Uncover the Hidden Illnesses

Lurking in Your Body

How to Reveal the Vibrant Youthful You

By Dr. Kirsten Ward

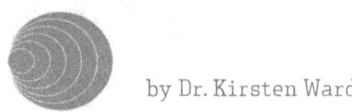

Personal Note from **Dr. Daniel Beilin, OMD, Lac** to my readers:

I applaud Kirsten for her drive and efforts to bring this technology (Alfa Thermometry) to the forefront and hope to establish its use in every major medical center worldwide. Kirsten Ward is one of the emerging experts in this field and it is a delight to see her taking the time to write a book which will help to educate Americans about this life-saving technique. She presents the history and theories to readers in an easy to understand way, and then she has shared with all of us her complete dissertation in the back of book which really digs into the medical jargon behind thermography.

This technology has helped to saved lives throughout the world and has a rich and long history, it should be embraced by our health system and a part of every person's yearly care routine.

I look forward to seeing what bright practitioners like Kirsten are doing for this area of healthcare and how it will grow and thrive in the future.

Wishing Health and Happiness for all of us…

Regards,

Dr. Daniel Beilin, OMD, LAc

Medical Director, Alfa Thermodiagnostics and the AlfaSight 9000 Regulation Thermometry Workstation. (www.alfa.global)

Editing and Layout: R.W. Jensen (solfire@phoenix-farm.com)

ISBN-13:978-1548915452
ISBN-10:1548915459

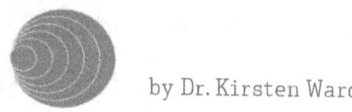

Dedicated to my wonderful family:

Harry, Britta and Oscar

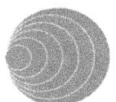

Table of Contents

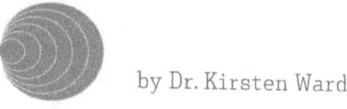

Chapter One:
Empowerment

Here is what you want and what you will get from this book: Empowerment over your own health and choices. We all want to live into our old age with as few aches and pains as we can manage. We want to be healthy and energetic, and certainly we hope to feel and look as young as possible for as long as possible. We all should be doing simple, easy and smart things now to ensure that we will grow old as gracefully as we can in our unique circumstances.

The big problem with our current health care system is that it treats all of us as if we are exactly the same, as if our bodies react exactly the same way to all medications and treatments. If you have struggled with not feeling well, but are just not satisfied with your diagnosis or current treatment, you need to reach out and see if one simple added therapy might be the answer to your long-term health challenges.

This book will lay out actual case studies (real stories/real people) as well as the scientific backing (this is FDA approved, by the way), and the long history of using thermography in order to treat your whole body and to help bring all the systems into line – similar to giving you a reboot on your health. The first case study is at the end of this chapter, placed here to show you a real person and a true medical plan with the real life reactions to that treatment. Then more case studies will follow throughout the book where that person's case study is connected with the topic being

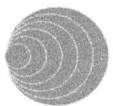

discussed – bringing to life the words on the page as they relate to real human beings.

So why empowerment? The flipside to encouraging our doctors and all health care professionals to realize we are not all the same, is that it takes a little longer to fish out what is really going on, and a little longer to fine-tune any treatments and lifestyle changes. The flipside for YOU is that you really have to engage, learn about yourself, your family's health history, AND you have to be willing to try something, decide if it works and stick with it – or decide that one new thing didn't work and research to find another treatment plan or another eating plan or another way to exercise ... you get the point.

Now, don't feel exhausted, once you put in the initial effort, you will only have to make very small adjustments to track your body's changes as you age, or change places where you live and work – to make sure things are not subtly changing and depressing the state of your health.

Your first step begins with this book: learn about thermography and the benefit it has been for countless people over the years. From there you can then figure out if and how it can be a help for you or a loved one. The case studies coming up will really help you to see how other people have suffered, then been treated and found relief – their real-life stories will put this all into perspective without medical and technical jargon words. I have written this book for you – not for other medical professionals – so I have tried to reach out to you, my readers, in a friendly tone, like we are talking over some coffee or tea. My credentials and my full dissertation are attached at the end for those of you who love to dig into the down and dirty details! I do, but I know many who will be reading this book won't have the time or even want to – but it is all there in the back this book for any of you who want MORE!

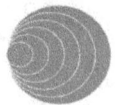

Learn to listen to the clues your body is giving you. As you learn, you become empowered when you choose which options you want to try in order to get back to optimum health.

This book is about the health care option called a thermogram – a thermogram is one of many diagnostic tools, just like an x-ray, an MRI, an ultrasound ... all tools used to take a deeper look at your body and what might be going on.

CASE STUDY #1

Person #1 is a 32 year old female who was suffering from severe fatigue. Her integrative doctor suspected Lyme's Disease. She did have mostly positive Lyme titers. Person #1 underwent her thermogram and it showed blocked areas in her sides and digestive track among other clues to internal systems that were struggling to function well. Due to her personal history and specific complaints and thermogram results, Person #1 was put on ozone therapy, sanum homeopathy, UVB exposure and parasite cleanse plans along with a detox plan specifically for her liver and kidneys. After four months, her follow up showed dramatic improvement in the lymphatic and intestinal blockages and she was able to resume a normal life after 4 years of sever fatigue.

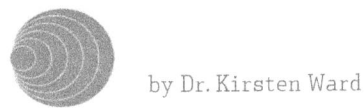

Chapter Two:
Thermogram Basics

What is a Thermogram?

A thermogram is diagnostic tool, like any tool a doctor uses. It looks beyond the skin deep symptoms and tries to find areas that are not working properly. Thermograms then take the next step to figure out how to fix what is going wrong. Just like an x-ray gives a picture of exactly where a bone may have fractured, a thermogram can give a picture of which internal organs are struggling to perform their jobs. Once you know which organs (or body systems) need more focused attention, that is when you can try some really specific treatment plans to get back to a healthy you.

Thermography is the discipline that uses a thermogram – like radiology is the discipline that uses x-rays. More specifically, thermography uses the heat patterns in your body to determine what is functioning normally and what is not by using temperature measurements connected with the time it takes the body to change temperatures in certain parts.

The best thing about a thermogram is you are NOT exposing your body to anything harmful; no x-rays, no drinking metallic chemicals – you can get them as often as you need to in order to keep track of (and on top of) changes. A small, hand-held ultra

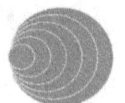

sensitive thermometer is used to take very strategically defined and placed measurements on specific areas of the skin (usually 120 different spots). These areas are related to the Chinese medical meridians as well as the dermatomes which are mapped by Western medicine. You can look up dermatome maps online and see how they are related to specific nerves and their journey through the brain and spinal cord to each and every part of the human body.

Currently, temperature readings are taken on 120 spots of the body. This gives your health care worker a baseline of where your body is functioning. Then all that happens next is your body is cooled down and the readings are taken again. Totally painless! This gives a measurement of how well your body is functioning by analyzing the work your body does to keep a steady core temperature.

The unique thing about a thermogram is it looks at functioning. Mammograms, x-rays and so forth give your care giver an idea of what is physically/structurally going on. This is certainly needed for things like bone fractures. Please understand that this book is NOT discounting these other medical diagnostic tools. However, some issues are not structural and for those issues a thermogram can be your best tool to find out what areas may be affecting your overall health.

Remember about the empowerment – and complexity issues. First you have to determine what the underlying cause or causes are of your illness or chronically feeling badly. Then you craft a plan of attack with your doctor and/or health care provider based on what you are finding out. I'll stress it one more time, this book is about the benefits of thermography, the reason for this book is to share with you knowledge about this under-used tool. So we are only delving deeply into this one subject, but it is not a reflection on the usefulness of other tools. Part of your empowerment is to listen to your body, read the clues it gives and use the tools that address those clues.

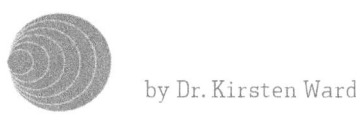

The Cool Down

After your baseline temperatures have been recorded, you will be put into a cool down phase – this is to provide your body a very slight stressor – but it is not super cold, and you will be in your underpants. The actual room will be a normal 70°F give or take – which is a normal room temperature.

What the light cold stressing is causing your body to do, is to respond by going into survival mode and moving your blood to the crucial parts of the body as biology sees it: your head and heart. Then the next readings are taken which show what systems are working normally and what systems may be sluggish or overactive in response to the cool air. Simple!

Who should get a Thermogram

Age

Thermograms are completely safe, no chemicals or other invasive issues. Technically they are safe for anyone. However, the thermogram is used to evaluate how body systems are functioning, and as such are ideally performed on bodies that are not very young and actively growing (like weeds). Normally the most accurate readings are obtained from people aged 12 and up. You are never too old to get more connected with your health.

CASE STUDY #2

Person #2 is a 70 year old male who was complaining of growing weakness. He had a history of aortic dissection, chronic mycosis and controlled hypertension. Person #2's thermogram showed lymph system blockage as well as immune stress and heavy metal indicators. He was put on a heavy metal detox, enzyme therapy and a liver detox. At his follow up thermogram Person #2 had renewed energy but also improved cardiac function. Below are two charts showing only two of over a hundred areas monitored at the start, one month and two month marks to illustrate the levels of improvement possible. Remember, as always, each person will be monitoring different areas closer than other areas and each person will have different levels of improvement over different time periods. We are all individuals.

Dental Issues

Anyone who has gum or dental issues should definitely schedule a thermogram. The connection of dental health and bacteria and viruses in the body is a well-established fact in the medical community. A thermogram can pick up issues in your gums and around your teeth that can be an early warning sign of serious issues with heart and blood heath, and therefore can give you a jumpstart on working back to health before more damage is done.

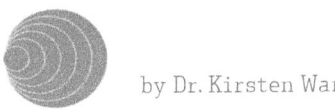

Other Requirements

Ideally, everyone should have a thermogram done as part of their yearly checkup. This provides a continual look at how a person's body may be changing. Because a body can still run – you can still be alive and working – but be functioning at a lower and lower level before it finally affects the structure of organs or bones ... having the thermogram can actually give you clues that something is wrong 8-10 years before a problem might trigger serious symptoms (as opposed to gentle clues) and show up on other diagnostic tests! So the bottom line on this is everyone should get a thermogram, but certainly at the first sign your body gives you that something is not right, you should have one and then monitor any changes.

Men and Women both benefit equally from a thermogram.

Exposure to certain viruses, bacteria, pollution and heavy metals can affect how your organs work. Anyone who is aware of having been exposed to these can benefit from a thermogram. Anyone who lives in a city will be constantly exposed to air pollution which is made of many different kinds of chemicals, depending on the region they live in and the types of production done in their area. A thermogram can help pinpoint if this exposure has affected any internal systems in your body.

Chronic fatigue is one of the most common symptoms that will indicate you could benefit from this treatment, followed by digestive issues. Both these conditions can have varied causes and often have interconnected causes – making them very complicated issues for other doctors to fully diagnose and/or treat.

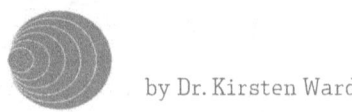

CASE STUDY #3

No personal statistics were permitted to be shared (age etc). Person #3 came in with no complaints to have a routine thermogram. The test results revealed chaotic regulation with severe multiple system blocks and a large temperature span over Person #3's entire body. Their physician referred #3 to an internist, Person #3 waited 4 months before eventually getting a CT Scan which revealed metastatic colon cancer.

The possible original causes may have been due to latent infections identified in the upper left dental area where the differences in adjacent teeth were over 2° - a full degree over normal differences in that area. It is well known that infections in the teeth or jaw can cause and certainly can contribute to many consequent diseases such as heart valve abnormalities.

Person #3 returned 5 months after the initial thermogram visit sharing the stage IV colon cancer diagnosis. They were to begin chemotherapy in a week. Working in concert with other health care providers – Person #3's organ systems were evaluated and the root cause was focused on during the treatment plan in conjunction with preparation by their natural health practitioner. The plan recommended was determined by what would work best with the other treatment plan. One focused on the very serious symptoms and the other one focused on the root cause.

Case Study #3 clearly shows the benefit of having routine thermographies done, as Person #3 had no symptoms going into the procedure.

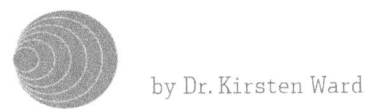

Chapter Three:
Back to Wellness

You have your thermogram results, now what?

Since this type of care focuses on the entire body as a functioning system with parts, your care provider will discuss the areas on your report that indicate they are working harder and come up with a plan with you. Wellness is like all things in life: a balance.

Your path to recovering your energy and good health will include learning about the systems in your body that are under extra stress. (Empowerment.) Then you will come up with a new eating plan (not a diet) and decide what building blocks your organ systems need. If you are not able to get all the nutrients for your body from your food, then the best types and brands of supplements will be discussed so that your body will be given all the raw material (vitamins, trace minerals) that it needs to start on its road to self-repair.

This author's position is that the body can make great strides to heal itself if you provide it with what it need. Controlling how you react to the high levels of stress that modern living puts on our mind and body is a key component. Because we explained earlier how each person has different conditions, changing even over their own lifetime; there can't be a list of recommendations that will work for all people. "Eat exactly this and take exactly that vitamin," simply will not be effective for everyone. Some people will need a raw food diet, some can stay on a fairly 'typical' diet and merely add trace minerals to their intake. Some people will need more vitamin C and so forth. In other words, you really need to have a thermogram of your specific condition and then drill down on the nutrients, exercises and other lifestyle conditions that help those organ systems that are showing they are in distress.

Stress was mentioned above, and it is a new kind of stress – one our bodies were not made to handle. Naturally, stress comes situationally and then goes away leaving peace until the next stressful situation. What I mean by this is that when hunting, running away from a lion, or other primitive situations, stress hit hard but then was over (one way or the other). In our lives that have gone from rural to cities with modern governments, people are now under constant stress and worry. Worry about finances, lease payments on cars or homes, keeping their jobs, constant noise and air pollution, fitting in socially ... you can see there are a wide variety of stressors that hit mentally as well as physically and they never ease up. We may not all be working out in the gym as much as we want to, but our bodies are constantly at war with how we have set up our lives.

This is a great drain on our bodies. Due to environment, our family history and genetics; each one of us will handle different incoming stress at a different efficiency level. And therefore a thermogram is so very important to look at YOUR body and what areas of your body will need a little more of a boost to keep functioning well.

Part of your plan back to wellness will be evaluating what stresses you, personally, are under in your life and adding ways to handle that stress to your other plans. When giving your body all of this wrapped up in one plan, your path back to wellness and energy and youth will be clear.

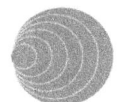

CASE STUDY #4

Person #4 was a 32 year old male when he came in for his thermogram. He suffered from anxiety and irritable bowel syndrome (IBS) as well as spontaneous sweating. He reported his body continuously felt hot. He shared his blood test results – which were normal. He was taking a prescription drug to help relieve his anxiety, but even so, reported intermittent periods of mental disorientation. If he simply was referred to a psychiatrist, he would likely be prescribed an accommodating or suppressive drug (just taking care of the symptoms) with no further investigation for a long term remedy. If the cause is not corrected, his anxiety may be controlled by drugs, but then he might suffer *other* symptoms as his body continues to breakdown from that original cause (dysfunction).

The questions for a comprehensive caregiving team should be:

1. What is the biological origin of the anxiety (central nervous system, gut, endocrine, insulin)?
2. Is the prescription drug causing complications such as worsening the IBS?
3. What are the possible causal factors of the IBS and anxiety (dental infection, metabolic abnormalities etc)?

Results of Person #4's thermogram looked first at the liver, pancreas and gut because those areas are usually functioning below normal standards when neurological disorders are the complaints. Part of the personalized assessment dealt with the medication he was on: it was possible the psychiatric drug was directly impacting his nervous system. Although the signature for heavy metal toxicity was found, investigation of the drug itself did not yield any information regarding this heavy metal poisoning suspicion. It could have been the drug or it could have been Person #4's own physiology causing the blockage of his systems. So, stimulation of the detoxification pathway by administering antioxidants, herbal liver therapy and certain enzymes were all part of the treatment plan.

Two months of being on this treatment plan a follow up thermogram was performed. Not only were the systemically blocked areas relieved, but 80% of the blockage was showing clear, normal and healthy self-regulation! Person #4 reduced his anti-anxiety prescription dosage by 50% and his gastrointestinal symptoms were reduced by nearly 80%! That was all in TWO MONTHS! (Note: normal positive signs show op around the 4 month mark.) All this improvement by treating the causes and not the symptoms.

Body Growth, Maintenance and Repair

My work toward gaining my doctorate was deeply concerned with this exact subject. I have added my full dissertation at the end of this book as Appendix One for those of you who want to dig into the scientific details. It contains some great history and citations of other works that can lead you on a deep research project if you are so inclined.

Most people don't have the time – or they roll their eyes when talking bio-chemical reactions – so I want to summarize here and offer the full work in Appendix One for those detail-loving people. So the following section will be a little more technical than the rest of the book – and you can get even *more* technical if you read the full paper at the end of the book if you like.

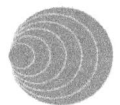

The body is always in a state of flux and change with the goal of maintaining a desired equilibrium; otherwise known as homeostasis. This is why tracking temperature changes can show us so much with a thermogram. When we look at a body trying to heal and readjust itself, what we see as "symptoms" are not necessarily something that needs fixing or repairing. We need to figure out what is going wrong – not the weakness, pain or other symptoms. Time and the body's own natural healing systems will take care of itself if given the proper support.

Meaning, YES, we need to notice symptoms – they are the clues our body is giving us that something is not working right. BUT, once we find out which body system or group of systems are struggling – we need to concentrate on them, making them healthier, giving them the nutrients they need – and the SYMPTOMS will actually go away on their own.

The reading of your report is connected to over 30 years of clinical research, it removed human subjectivity errors in the analysis of your body's functioning and presents usually the top 6 imbalances in your body (there are over 40 different types that are evaluated for disease and dysfunction.) The sensitivity of the test allows for a dysfunction to be observed up to 8-10 years before structural changes in the tissues are visible. Targeted preventative measures can then be decided upon to address these dysfunctions before structural changes become harder to correct.

According to Lutz and Mazzur, disease can be prevented "on three levels: primary, secondary and tertiary." (Lutz, 2015) At the primary prevention level the goal is to "avert the occurrence of disease." The secondary prevention level is designed to utilize "monitoring techniques to discover incipient diseases early enough to enhance the opportunity to control their effects." The tertiary prevention level is where nutrition is used as a treatment "after a disease has occurred

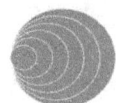

to prevent complications or to promote maximum adaptation." The common thread at every one of these levels of prevention is the application of principles of nutrition that optimize individual body healing.

To date it has been discovered that the body requires approximately 50 essential factors that must come from our environment. These include: 20 or 21 minerals, 13 vitamins, 9 essential amino acids, 2 essential fatty acids, 2 types of fiber, water, oxygen, light and a source of energy (usually starch or glucose). Drinking lots of good quality water, consuming high quality foods with dense nutrients, exposing the skin to sunlight in a healthy way and breathing lots of clean air, is the best way to achieve a good quality of life. Living in today's world, most of the individuals I have crossed paths with have suffered with compromised digestive tracts that negatively impact the goal of having a good quality of life.

The great thing about my practice is that I share your report and plan with your primary care doctor, and if that doctor is not familiar with thermography, I offer a *free* 15 minute phone consultation with your doctor so that ALL of your health care steps are working together. This is a process and we embrace all the tools that will help us on our path back to wellness.

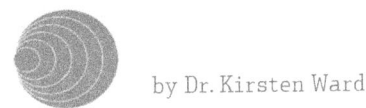

Chapter Four:
My Early Life & Marriage

I was born in Germany to German parents. Both parents were from Post WW II Germany and both survived the rebuilding with scant health care and the general stresses of war-torn Germany. My mother came to West Germany at 17, after having been stuck behind the Iron Curtain in what was former East Prussia. This was the first time she saw a banana, a telephone and her father! My father grew up in the industrial city of Düsseldorf. He would tell tales of catching a ride on an ocean freighter and riding up the Rhein River only to be carried by the current back downstream.

I was born in Düsseldorf. When I was an infant, the doctors informed my parents that my hips were not fully formed. Basically, I was dysplastic. As treatment for this condition, the doctors back then would place the baby on their back in a cast where the legs were suspended and anchored to each side of the crib. This is how I slept until my parents made the move to the United States when I was 18 months old.

Before we made the move across the ocean I suffered with febrile convulsions. My parents spared no expense making sure I recovered and that there were no permanent effects on my growing body. All the test results from my extensive health care history were written in German. When we got to the United States, my mother looked for a pediatrician who could read and understand the results. She finally found one. My new pediatrician prescribed Phenol Barbitol preventatively. This

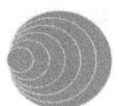

disrupted my sleep and my mother would later describe finding me asleep under lamps with my blanket. She attributed this to the medication. Of course, at this point we were not able to verify or dispute this cause and effect. Suffice it to say I had disrupted sleep patterns as a child. Additionally, I had multiple ear infections and other needs for which I was given rounds of antibiotics. All my childhood immunizations were brought up to date. The only unusual characteristic of my childhood immunizations compared to a typical child of that era was that I was given purple juice for Polio. The pediatrician wanted to make sure that I did not have another seizure by spacing the doses out. Her intentions resulted in success in this area. I didn't have another seizure as a small child.

Recollections of my early childhood were pleasant. I played in the sunshine and in the dirt. At 3 I was joined by a younger sister. She was the picky one of the family, and persuaded my father to start smoking outside the home instead of inside.

When I was 6 my father was transferred to Sao Paulo, Brazil. In the middle of the school year and a Chicago blizzard, my mother took my sister and me to join my father in Brazil. I was enrolled in a German-speaking private school. Luckily, my parents had insisted that I learn German in Chicago to keep close to my German roots. My classmates in Brazil spoke varying degrees of German, but absolutely no English. Talk about stress!

The social life of a kid in Brazil was very different from that in the United States. Those kids did not play with other kids, but they played with their maids. My mother had the unenviable task of entertaining my younger sister while I was at school. The bus would pick me up while it was still dark outside. I remember imitating my father by pretending to be smoking in the cool morning.

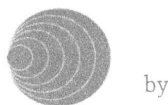

We were living in a two-bedroom apartment. We would walk to the grocery store and en route we played in the sandboxes. Unbeknownst to us, those sandboxes were not for humans to play in. They were for the animals to use. That explained the number of small bug bites on us in the morning: fleas and other insect bites.

The destitute were very numerous in 1970s Brazil. There was a time when my mother, sister and I were walking home from the grocery store together. My sister was so excited to have been able to purchase a flavored yogurt dessert that she was carrying it with the swagger only a 3 year-old could pull off. Coming towards us was a very pregnant woman with a young child in tow. She began talking to my mother in Portuguese. My mother had not yet learned to speak Portuguese and kept repeating the phrase, "I don't understand." This did not deter the woman. She kept pointing to my sister and the yogurt she was holding. This back and forth went on for what seemed like an hour to a young me. Most likely it was only a few minutes. That was the last time my sister carried a treasure home from the store that other people could see.

On the health front, I was frequently unable to keep my breakfast down. I began to vomit the orange juice I would drink for breakfast. My mother switched me from eating cream of wheat to French toast. Apparently, many of the boxes of cream of wheat contained insects as you would expect in those years from living in a tropical climate. I also continued to have fitful sleep patterns. I was a fearful child and would have frequent nightmares. Thus began my mind game of leaving or placing "ghosts" in my old bedroom and starting fresh in the new bedroom. Luckily, we moved frequently and I would leave these bad thoughts behind.

For our stay in Brazil, my father's passport was stamped with a requirement to receive an immunization for something. For an unknown reason my mother's, my sister's and my passports did

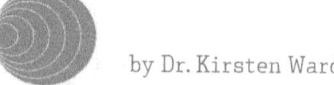

not have this same requirement. We all went to have this immunization anyway. It went something like this: we waited in line with all these other Brazilians. There was a man in a uniform who had an air-gun like contraption. Once you got to the front of the line you would pull your sleeve up over your shoulder. The uniformed man would aim the air-gun at your arm, there would be a little poof sound and then you could move out of the way to make room for the next person in line. It didn't feel like a shot, or even hurt. There was just a little bit of pressure. But I will tell you what ... that evening you couldn't raise your arms parallel to the ground. It was very sore. So even though all of us were not required to get this immunization, we all did. To this day, I am not sure what it was for.

One other event that I remember with fondness was a time we went to visit some of my father's colleagues. We were sitting in the yard underneath banana and coconut trees. All of us children were running around the yard with abandon. It was a pleasant day. Discussion turned to bugs ... again. This time it was for a particular bug that would lay eggs just under the skin of the human host. The egg mass would mature and then finally burst through the skin to release the next generation of insects into the world and the host would be left with a gaping hole in the skin until the body healed itself. It was so gross that of course this is what stuck in the memory of a young girl.

Another memory I have of Brazil is birthday parties. Since most of my classmates were living in Sao Paulo proper, they were also in apartments. Playing party games in an apartment was tricky. So, we would go to the parking garages that were underneath the buildings and locked away from everyday passersby. A very popular game was Hit the Bucket. We were blindfolded, spun slowly around in a circle and then given a wooden spoon. The idea was to hit the ground with the wooden spoon until the bucket was found. If we found the bucket with

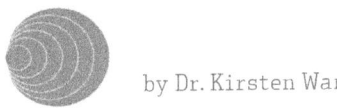

the spoon, then we could keep the treasure that was hidden underneath it. All this fun in a parking garage. It was active and in the outdoors – true childhood fun with face to face socializing.

As any child does, I was working at acclimating myself to this new and exciting environment of Brazil. Suddenly one day, we received notification that my mother's father had passed away in Germany. At the same time my father's boss was found dead of a heart attack. With the death in my mother's family and the loss of support for my father's career, my father decided that we needed to pack up and leave Brazil. The wrinkle came when we tried to leave Brazil. Apparently, the snag happened because of the immunizations that we all received, but that only my father was required to have. Bureaucracy and red tape is a great way to frustrate people. My father had to perform a magic trick, as only a father could, in order for us to have been allowed to leave the country after such a misstep.

As a kid, all I remember of this time period is that we moved in with my mother's family and slept on the floor of my grandmother's suite (she was on the second floor of a multi-generational house in Germany). I went to school with my cousin, my sister was paired up with a neighborhood boy who was also in Kindergarten. From my memory, this seemed to last a few months. I made quite a few new friends in the town and my German was getting better all the time. During school recess, I was frequently asked to count to 100 in English. I was also asked to participate in the classroom. One of the teacher's favorite activities was to have an alphabet board on the wall. She would spell out words, one letter at a time, and expect us to know what the word was. Even though I was an avid reader, I never was successful at deciphering the English words she spelled out for us. Was this stress? I don't know. I do know that I was just as frustrated as the teacher was by the end of the day.

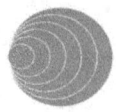

Not too long after this we returned to the U.S. and moved to Pennsylvania. Boy was I happy to get back to familiarity. We lived in an apartment outside of Pittsburg. I went into the 2nd grade. I remember looking at the 1976 bicentennial quarters that were all over the place. A whole gang of us kids built a fort out of scavenged trash in a nearby wooded area. We would spend hours in the woods perfecting our hideout. After finishing out the year there, we moved back to the Chicago metropolitan area.

Things were stable from 3rd through the middle of 7th grade. I went to school with the same neighborhood kids and felt secure. German was not offered at my school, so I opted for French. Private German schooling happened once a week (usually Friday evenings). This cut into my sleepover schedule with friends, but it was non-negotiable to my parents so I had no choice.

My sister had always wanted a pet, so my parents found a chocolate lab breeder in the area. We drove out to the house to pick out this wonderful, small, male puppy. I remember being afraid of his sharp little teeth. He lasted 24 hours before my parents decided it was too much trouble for us and returned him back to the breeder. My fear of dogs began at that point.

When I was about 12 we were vacationing in Florida. My father had a friend who had an apartment on Sanibel Island before anything else was built up on the island. We would often spend Thanksgiving there, since we had no other family to go to. My mother never did master the art of cooking a turkey and so making her famous duck or goose with Knödel was always an entire. all-hands-on-deck family affair.

During one trip that I remember, we were visiting the Thomas Edison home. Visitors were given access to all the buildings. We were standing in his laboratory filled with vials, flasks and other chemistry contraptions when I had a most unusual

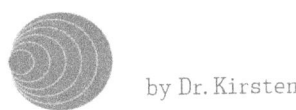

feeling. I turned to my father and asked him if we could leave. He said something about the tour not being over and that I would not have long to wait. The next thing I knew all these people were standing around me and I was looking up at them. I had passed out. After a few moments I felt well enough to get up. The vacation continued without any other events that I remember. We don't know the cause of the blackout, but this was the first time I went totally down to the ground. There were other frequent light-headed episodes. If I got up from a seated position too quickly, I would often have to hold onto a table and focus on not going down again as the periphery of my vision began to go black. When we asked the doctor about these episodes I was told to drink coffee and eat sugar or salt to help increase my blood pressure.

When I had my first menstrual cycle I started having extreme PMS issues. Bloating, cramping, all the discomforts you can imagine. Most challenging to my family, however, was my mood. About 3-4 days before my period would begin I would be having an emotional meltdown - lots of tears. There was not much that could be done to help me at that point. I just had to cry myself out.

One day at school someone came into my science class and told me that my name was on a list on the office door. I was mortified. Why was my name on this list? What did I do to get into some kind of trouble? I was too nervous to even go and look. Luckily someone clarified that it was the Honor Roll. Of course, she had to explain exactly what the Honor Roll was, since I had never heard of such a thing. Then, the third quarter of 7th grade my parents moved us again. This time we were moving from a suburb of Chicago to one of the top 10 preppy towns in the United States - Darien, Connecticut. I had no idea what was in store for me.

For me, growing up a day in Chicago looked like this: I shared a small locker with another girl. The school was filled to

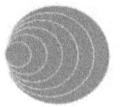

bursting with a rainbow of ethnicities. We had PE every day. Showers were required. The girls would line up single file with not a stitch of clothing on. We would snake into the shower room in single file and then snake out again, in single file. Just outside the shower room the PE teachers would be standing with a clip board. We would give them our number that was marked off on a list on that clip board. In exchange, we would be given a towel that was 2' x 3' and less than 5 minutes to change in preparation for the bell to ring for the next class. We had 50 minute classes that met every day.

Now came Darien: we had a 7-day rotating schedule. Each day one class fell off to allow the other classes to be lengthened. This meant that every morning the first question was: "What day is it today, A, B, C, D, E, F, G?" PE met a couple of times during that rotation – but not every day. No one took showers during school, but then we never really worked hard enough to need one. That first semester in Darien (they worked on 2 semesters not quarters) it turned out that I was so far behind in French class that I had to go for remedial help almost every morning to get me up to speed. I ended up having 5 quarters worth of grades that year. As for ethnicity: we had one building that housed the ABC girls (A Better Chance in Darien ... they were the five or six hand-picked top African American kids in their home schools. They were given the opportunity to live in a house together – usually girls – with some teacher chaperones; when a Japanese family moved into our neighborhood the house was spray painted with "Go home" and "Kamikaze." Otherwise British Protestant churches populated the town. Being Lutheran we went to a church in a neighboring town. There were only a smattering of Germans in the area.

Girls did not carry purses or wear makeup in Darien. All were considered beautiful in their natural state. This was very different from what I had experienced in Chicago.

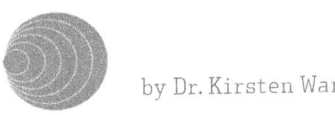

This was also the first time I was truly bullied. There were a couple of girls who would throw supplies at me during art class. As they were throwing things at me they were claiming that I had killed their relatives back in Europe. Since I had only lived in Germany until I was 18 months old, I'm not quite sure how they came to their logical conclusion, but there was no opportunity to talk to them. The teacher had no control of the class, so this ended up being my least favorite class of the day.

My luck would change soon. We were the last 9th grade class to leave that middle school. Due to lack of students, the middle school I was attending was going to be repurposed for government offices. With the combining of my middle school and the other school in town there were a whole lot of kids who were new to each other. This was an opportunity to meet more people. Plus, when the 8th and 9th graders moved into the high school together I was no longer one of the Freshman. I was already a Sophomore. This was the year I took biology. It was my favorite subject. They even called me Dr. Lorenz because my classmates were convinced that I was going to be a doctor when I grew up. So it seems my scientific research skills started early.

As with other girls my age this was the time when body image became important to me. I began the yo-yo dieting that was so common then. Exercise classes and a variety of diet methods were cycled through by all of us girls. My weight would go up and down, depending on a variety of causes.

I filled up most of my free time with as many activities as I could. I participated in Peer Tutoring training, Debate Club, German School, Piano lessons, Confirmation class just to name a few. Since I wasn't tuned in to the resume-padding or other things people did to get into good colleges, I was driven purely by my own interests.

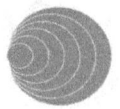

Darien High School was one of the first schools to offer the International Baccalaureate (IB) in the United States. Since I had German citizenship, and would have the opportunity to go to Germany to attend the universities there at no charge, I decided to look into the program. There were a number of elements that the IB required that were not covered by the regular curriculum. For this I had to return to school for night classes a couple of times a week. These were the most fun for me. We discussed non-Euclidian geometry, logical thinking, the great books course and comparative religions. I looked forward to listening to the heated discussions that happened in these afterschool classes.

But listen is all that I could do. I had clammed up totally in school. It was a rare day when I spoke up at all until many years later. I did not feel comfortable sharing my experiences. Looking back on it I realize that my contributions would have been great since they were so different from anyone else's, but at the time you couldn't have convinced me of that. During my graduation party Jonathan Karl (the ABC News reporter) came up to me at a party holding out his hand and introducing himself to me. I quickly informed him that I had been in the same English class with him for the entire year. Obviously, I was that invisible. This invisibility made me feel safe, while at the same time making it difficult for others to get to know me.

There was another activity in English class where we were to have written poems and then they were anonymously read out by others in the room. I remember when they read my poem; those who were discussing it insisted it was this other student's writing. He corrected them, but they still attributed the writing to him. I said not a word.

One of the things that used to trouble me the most was the Pledge of Allegiance. I was a German citizen who had been brought to the United States by my parents. While I loved it

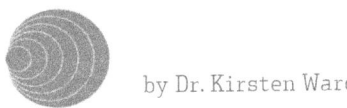

here and considered it my home, I was not going to be able to vote. Getting into any kind of trouble might have resulted in deportation – not a desirable outcome. At least that's the way it was in my teenager mind. So, since it was required to stand and recite the pledge, I would stand and mumble something. It was very uncomfortable for me.

One summer we had spent, what I considered, an extremely long time in Germany. I was homesick for my own familiar surroundings in the United States. While we were waiting at the German airport two military police came and questioned me. They kept asking if I was really the daughter of these two adults that were sitting near me - my actual parents. I was totally freaked out. All that I could think about was, "I am sure as hell going home and you can't make me stay here one more day." To this day, I am not sure what it was all about.

I had to admit defeat when it came to completing the requirements for the IB. There were too many small, missing elements for me to fit into my already full schedule. Instead I focused on my German Staats Examen I and II (tests given by the German government to verify language abilities sufficient to attend the universities in Germany) and AP exams. It ended up that Vanderbilt gave me 12 credit hours (4 classes) for my efforts. That was quite a bit for that day and age – especially for a private college. Additionally, the Staats Examen I and II together with 4 semesters at Vanderbilt qualified me for the Abitur (the German equivalent of the IB), and opened the door of finishing college in Germany if I wanted.

Since neither of my parents had attended college, I needed to navigate that on my own, all new territory. My high school had an over 95% college attendance rate, so help was available if only I asked. My guidance counselor was instrumental in helping me navigate my way through all the choices. We narrowed it down to about 5 schools. That was considered a lot of schools at that time: 1 early decision, 1 safety and 1 reach

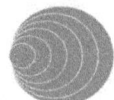

was the norm. In the end, the choice was easy: Vanderbilt University was the only school that accepted me.

I had become somewhat defiant of my parents' influence over me and I insisted on writing my college essay without their help. The essay that got me into college focused on all the interpersonal skills that I had developed doing peer tutoring activities and other volunteer activities. My father was always perplexed that I would "work for free" at my volunteer jobs. But in this case my defiance paid off. It was thanks to these efforts that I had the experiences to write an acceptance worthy essay.

My Senior year was a blur. Alex Kelly (See People Magazine vol. 46 #19) was given a diploma in the middle of the year to not show up in school any more, senior slump hit, and I knew I was going to Vanderbilt University no matter what. Everything seemed to be going well but a tragedy hit. One of my circle of friends was killed on the way home from finals. There were 5 people in the car. The driver got off without a scratch, but the girl in the seat behind him was crushed into a telephone pole on the way home, in the middle of the day. There was no foul play, but the driver couldn't make the turn and the back end of the car found the middle of the telephone pole. The girl in the middle of the seat in the back was badly injured. No one else sustained more than a few scratches. This was devastating for a small school. We were given time off to go to the funeral. It was during the day.

It was the second funeral I had attended that year. I had been working at a farmer's market in Darien when one of the two owners was on his way back from New York City with produce when he was cut off on the road. His van flipped and he was pronounced dead at the scene. Those were two eye-opening experiences for me. I had not been given the opportunity to really experience my grandparents aging and these were both people in the prime of their lives. It was like a slap in the face.

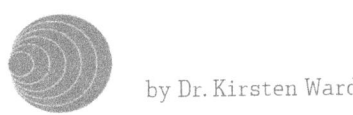

It changed my mental outlook. Maybe I would be next. No time to waste. I needed to live life to the fullest since it could be over in a flash.

That summer I was going to Institute Villa Pierre-Feu for the summer. Institute Villa Pierre-Feu is an international Finishing School and one of the few left in the world. I was told that I was the first American they ever let attend. Of course, I was German, not American (North American for all my South and Central American classmates). My first experience was getting picked up at the train station. I was picked up by a private car. The car broke down half way around Lake Geneva on the way to the school. I remember the driver begging me to explain the car problems to the mistress of the school. I was clueless about why this even could be a big deal. After all, no one was hurt and I finally arrived. When he safely deposited me at the front door, I was greeted by this fireball of a woman who quickly accosted me with the question, "Did you not know that we sent someone to pick you up?" I had no comments to this, but the driver came in and took over the apologies. I was free to find my own way around.

This was my first adventure into an all-female environment. I took my job as ambassador of the United States very seriously. All the girls were curious about my life. And I was curious about theirs. My roommates were from Punjab and from Kuwait. The girl from Punjab had arrived before me, but her luggage did not. We pitched in and let her wear some of our clothes until her trunk arrived. Unfortunately, her trunk arrived complete with all her winter clothes and the moth balls they were packaged with.

On the first night, my Punjabi roommate was hungry so we went to the kitchen in search of a snack. The only person on duty was an elderly lady who spoke only French. I had had a few years of French in high school, but my roommate had not had any, so communication was a challenge. The lady offered us some fruit.

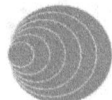

My roommate took a banana and thanked her for it. As we turned to leave the woman came running after us with a plate, fork and knife in hand. We assured her, as anyone who could only speak a few words in the language, that we were only going to eat the banana. We didn't need a plate, fork and knife to do that. Only after our classes started and we learned how to eat the banana with a fork and knife, did that encounter make more sense. That woman was giving us the necessary utensils to eat the snack she offered. Looking back on the event reminds me of the Seinfeld episode where everyone was eating chocolate bars with a fork and knife.

The entire time I was at this school my head was pounding. The headache was terrible. I am not sure of the origin, but when I left the school the headache went with it. Others who claimed to have this same problem blamed it on the altitude. That is a definite possibility. I have frequently struggled with altitude issues since then.

We cooked all our own meals (under the direction of the cooking instructor), we learned how to arrange flowers, serve guests, direct domestic help and all assortment of lessons geared towards helping us understand international cultural and protocol. It was a memorable summer.

Vanderbilt was a tough transition for me. There were 4 of us attending from my high school. Two with dual citizenship and two "typical" Darien people. Southern culture was challenging for me. It was so foreign: people paid fraternities and sororities to be their friends and interactions that happened face to face were vastly different from those that happened when there was a turned back. Additionally, the only wars my family ever talked about were WW I and WW II. Nashville had few northerners and was still fighting Civil War battles. One of the debates that continually astounded me was the one about whether Texas counted as a southern state. All those who lived in the former Confederate states claimed that Texas was not a

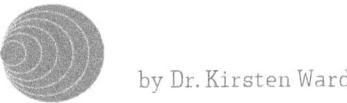

true participant in the Civil War and therefore could not be considered a part of the southern states. Texans, on the other hand, were steadfast in their belief that they were. I would just listen to them in amazement.

The summer after my Freshman college year I went to Hurricane Island Outward Bound for a 64-Semester course on the coast of Maine. This course was accepted at some colleges for credits (of course Vanderbilt was not one of those schools). We were put through a standard 21-day sailing course and then put through several leadership challenges. For the entire 64-days we slept out in the elements. Sometimes on a platform tent and other times on the sailing vessel, and still other times in camping tents: I was in heaven.

AIDS was big in the news that summer. Early reports suggested that mosquitoes might be transmitting the disease from one person to another. We were outside, in Maine ... there were plenty of mosquitoes as well as black flies and no-see-ums (little bitters!). I resigned myself to thinking that I just might get AIDS. Of course, transmission like this has not ever been substantiated.

One day we were all participating in a silent hike. Not sure what possessed me, but I jumped off a boulder directly into a crevice. My ankle twisted. It was a pretty bad sprain. The choice given to me was that either I complete the course or go home now. Well, I was not going to bow out. I was too happy with all that I was experiencing. I decided to persevere. One of the participants knew just what to do with a sprained ankle and would help me tape it up in the mornings. This let me keep going in the course.

Outward Bound is where I was exposed to Kurt Hahn and the educational philosophy of using nature and challenges to teach life lessons. This is also where I encountered vegetarianism and Michio Kushi for the first time.

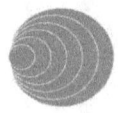

At the end of the course I went back to Vanderbilt. It was a hard transition back. Being in the supportive and encouraging environment of Outward Bound I felt stifled in the southern university setting. I was ready to do something with my life. I decided to try my hand at college in Germany. I kept up my daily running (still on a fragile ankle) and the vegetarian diet I recently started. When I arrived back at school I could sleep on the floor in the middle of a room full of people and not hear a thing. My fitful sleep patterns from childhood had finally gone away.

During my Freshman year, I had made friends with a girl from Florida. We began living in the French hall in the foreign language dormitory during our Sophomore year. I decided to take the highest-level physics I could, since I had decided I was going to make the transition to Germany the following fall. My thinking was based on the fact that everyone at the universities in Germany had completed a year of high school physics. I had not done that. Since I only had a single semester left before I was going to leave, I chose to challenge myself in the upper level course, one designed for engineering and science majors. This did not end well for me. The professor was a very nice man. When I went to him right before the drop/add period was over he told me to hang in there for the next test and decide after that. Well, I scored something like 25/200 with 20 points for putting my name on the paper. I could no longer drop the class, so I just stopped going. I had to repeat this same class to have the grade replaced with a better one. Summer school, here I come.

Summer school was much less stressful than the school year. I was living in a building that should have been condemned, but was full of college kids. There was no A/C and we hit over 100 degrees in Nashville that summer. I spent most of my time reading, cross stitching and studying physics. That is, until I met a boy. We hit it off right away, but there were only a few

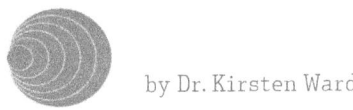

weeks of summer school left ... and I was not coming back in the fall. I would be in Germany.

I went to Germany where I started off my transition with an internship at a huge conglomerate. I was placed in a department where I spent the entire day looking up data and rewriting it into spreadsheets. After that was completed I advanced to reformatting the forms in their heavy-duty printer. All the while I was living with my grandmother. On weekends, I would go and visit the girls I had met in Switzerland. I lived for the weekends. During the work week I shared the top floor of the office building with three middle-aged smokers and one girl my age who carried a concealed handgun in a country that did not allow guns. On the weekends, I would visit the girls and spend time doing the things teenage girls did. We went shopping, cooking and found general entertainment.

While living with my grandmother, I applied to the university programs. I also had to find a place to live. This was a tough proposition. For one apartment, I showed up with 15 other girls and the place was a mess. There were pieces of wood hanging down from the ceiling and sheet rock disintegrating onto the broken-up floor. The landlady said that we would need to fix it up before we moved in. I went to visit a few other places, but the situations were similar. Not something a little bit of paint would fix, rather what was needed was totally new flooring and repairing falling beams, etc. This was a bit out of my repair comfort zone.

I was also still receiving letters from the boy back in the US. It was time to begin the process of going back to finish up at Vanderbilt. The trick was going to be to figure out how to graduate on time. I had changed my major several times and wasn't too sure about any of them. When I got back to school the counselor and I discovered that I could finish on time if I completed an interdisciplinary degree. That meant a lot of the introductory courses I tried wouldn't count toward my major,

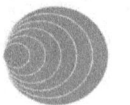

but I could complete the upper level courses in those disciplines and still graduate on time. Thank goodness I had gotten credit for all those courses from high school. European Studies here I come.

I completed my BA. I now had two choices: either I could support myself entirely on my own, or I could continue to go to school. Knowing the kind of jobs my classmates were landing, or rather not landing, I opted to go back to school. Vanderbilt was connected with Peabody College which was for teachers. I applied and was accepted. Since I had the interdisciplinary undergraduate degree, they strongly suggested that I try and get as many endorsements as I could to be more marketable. I opted to go back and get a history and a German major. Graduate school took an additional two years with one entire semester of student teaching. I taught German at a magnet school in downtown Nashville. Turns out that one of my students was the son of the professor I had for that physics class that I had stopped attending. He was part of an exceptionally brilliant class of students. The world is a small and wonderful place.

When I went to the beach for a short break, I decided not to put sunscreen on the back of my legs in order to let them get a bit of color and thereby look smaller. Here was my self-image problem coming out again. Unfortunately, I let my legs get a little bit too sunburned. They swelled up. When we finally got out of the sun and into the room, I passed out in the shower and hurt my foot and leg. Luckily, I got help getting out of the shower. I spent half the day in bed sleeping off the stress of that event. There was no way that I was going to the hospital or doctor. I hobbled around a few days on a sprained foot. The sunburn did a nice peel.

Turns out that the boy I met while repeating physics is the one I decided to marry after college. Typically, the bride is the one who determines which church hosts the wedding. In my case, the pastor that had confirmed me was forcibly retired because it

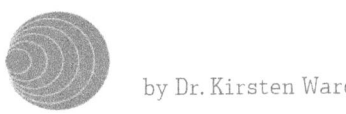

came out that he had molested children when he was at a different church. My future husband's family had been at their church for generations, and we were going to get married in the chapel that was donated by one of our classmates at Vanderbilt. That was good enough for my parents. The only down side was that my German relatives struggled with pronouncing Presbyterian. After all, Germans are historically either Lutheran or Catholic. In the end, my sister's godfather was the only family member to make it from Germany. Most of those who came to the wedding were from my husband's family.

We were married 4 years before we decided to have children. We had both been working in Houston for the steel industry at decent jobs. We would frequently talk about business outside of work hours and now decided to branch out into family time. We were working for competitors, but they were friendly competitors. The lower end of his customer base was the upper end of ours. It was a stable time in our lives. We had also taken parenting for a trial run. First, we had a cat and then added a dog to our little family. Those were adjustments for me, since we had grown up without pets. I really loved, and still do love, all of my critters.

When we decided to have a baby, we were both as ready as could be. We were going on vacation in Taos, New Mexico. One of our first real vacations. His parents were meeting us there for a couple of days. The doctors advised us not to announce the pregnancy, since the first trimester is a challenging time for new mothers and babies and that is typically the time when a miscarriage might occur. When we showed up in Taos his father had left me an issue of The Atlantic Monthly which showcased many studies about the fertility rate decline in older women. It was an inside joke that we were already pregnant but couldn't say anything.

Carrying a baby to term in the heat of Houston was challenging. I ballooned to over 200 lbs with the pregnancy and had

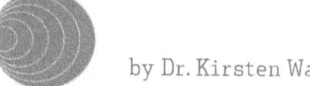

frequent swollen feet. I had a lot of trouble being out in the heat. It was difficult to do much. I had already given notice at work that I wasn't going to come back, so I was able to relax right before the event. The due date for the delivery came. As the day went on, I kept having a weird feeling. I took a nap and after I woke up my husband and I decided it would be a good idea to call the doctor. He immediately sent us in to the hospital. On our way to the hospital we bought batteries for the camera (no smartphones then) and made plans to go to a local car show afterwards. We never left the hospital that night. It turns out that my water had broken.

Based on my bodies clues that morning (the weird feelings) my doctor declared that it had probably broken in the morning. At that time, it was believed that the baby needed to be born 24 hours after the water had broken to minimize any other problems. The doctor explained to me that since I had not even gone into labor yet, let alone had the baby drop, they were going to induce labor and that I was looking at about 20 hours of labor. Turns out I was in for only 5 hours of labor. My beautiful daughter was born just before midnight on the day she had been due. She was a big baby (coming in at 9 lbs, 2 oz.) and got stuck in the birth canal. This resulted in a bit of stiffness in her right side. The Houston medical community had a policy that they removed all newborns for 6 hours of observation after birth. So, promptly at 6am I started asking the nurses to bring me my baby. However, it wasn't until 8am that they brought her to me. My mother made the trip down from Connecticut and my mother-in-law came in from Fort Worth. They met in the bathroom before heading into the room where my husband, my baby and I were napping.

My daughter was a colicky baby. I nursed her and found it was better for her if I ate chicken, green beans and potatoes. Much of anything else and she would have problems. When she was 3 months old she spiked a fever. We took her to the hospital and they determined that she had a urinary tract infection from a

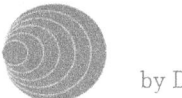

calcium deposit. The mother's milk I gave her calcified in her system. Treatment for this was IV antibiotics. She and I were in the hospital for 3 days together. I never left her side. Her colic continued. Now it was accompanied by yeast infections and diaper rashes and ear infections. When she was 11 months old I weaned her and she went straight to a cup.

At this time, several things happened in quick succession: I found out I was pregnant again, we began the move to the Chicago area and my college roommate was diagnosed with breast cancer soon after she started her full-time job as a mergers and acquisition attorney.

My college roommate's cancer diagnosis was unusual. She was so young that the medical community had difficulty giving her recommendations. She attempted to persuade them into letting her have a radical mastectomy, but the rule at the time was tissue preservation and they denied her request. About a year later she had another round of cancer in the other breast. About a year after that they found more in the first breast. Not too long after that there was a tumor in her brain. She lost her battle around the time she would have been 30. Here was another reminder for me to enjoy every moment of life.

My family of 3½ moved to the Chicago area. We ended up in a small neighborhood where there were lots of kids. After my second child was born, I struggled with post partum depression. I was sleep deprived: he was a hungry baby, eating every 1.5 - 2 hours 24 hours a day; my daughter was teething and would spend nights crying out in pain; I was working full time with an hour commute each way. I had to leave the job and work on getting through this tough time. Once out of the darkness I went back to work.

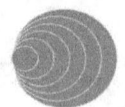

This neighborhood was a great place for all the kids. There was a gang of about 12 of them ranging in age from 12 down to 3 years old. We would have impromptu block parties with kids running up and down the street. I was working at a tool steel company and my husband was still working for the bigger steel company, those were wonderful times.

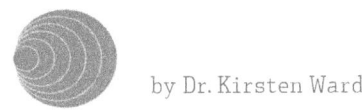

Chapter Five:
My Family Health & Behavior Challenges

My daughter was showing continued signs of struggling as she grew. She was screened to join a special group within a daycare that focused on school preparedness because she was "at risk" of school failure. We knew that certain things were challenging for her, but were not sure what was tipping her over the edge. There was no consistency or pattern to her behavior that we could see. My second child who was only 22 months younger displayed none of these struggles.

One morning I came down with something (the kids were constantly bringing illnesses into the house so we were frequently fighting something off). I woke up in the morning to get ready for work. Standing in the kitchen I passed out and broke a glass of water on the floor. This time my husband insisted that I go to the hospital. Turns out I was dehydrated and they gave me IV fluids and sent me home. My daughter was pretty shaken up because she came into the kitchen and saw me on the floor. I was unable to get up. Just a little hiccup in the journey, but a life lesson that something as simple as being dehydrated can go unnoticed if you don't pay attention to the clues you body is giving you. I could have saved my daughter that fear and myself those hours in the hospital just by drinking a glass of water a few hours earlier.

My daughter's behavior was being addressed at school, my son was enjoying his time at school, my husband and I were working.

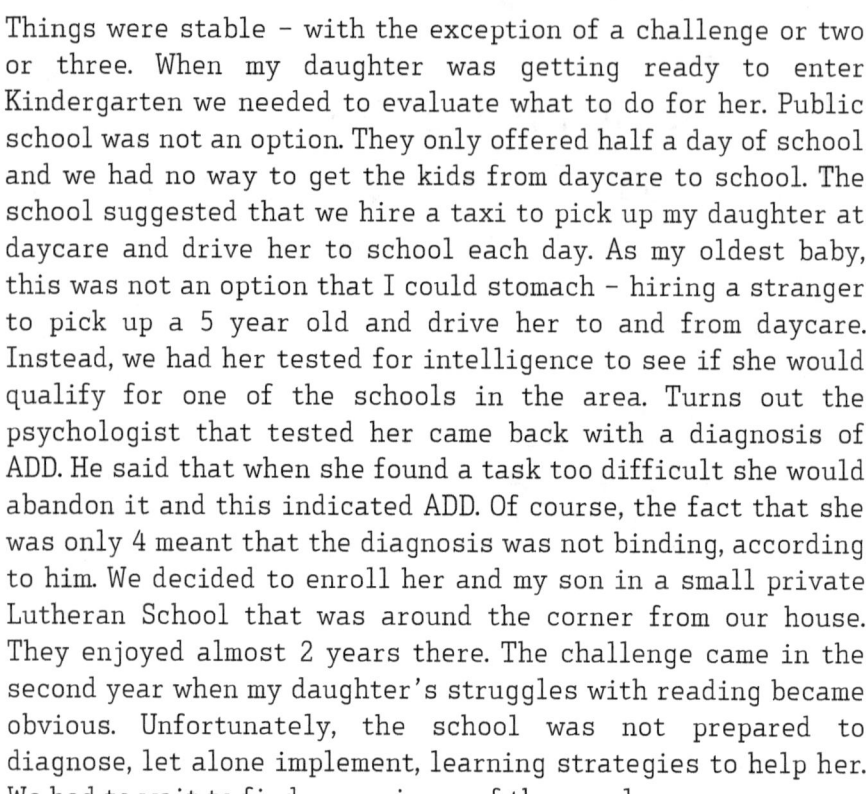

Things were stable – with the exception of a challenge or two or three. When my daughter was getting ready to enter Kindergarten we needed to evaluate what to do for her. Public school was not an option. They only offered half a day of school and we had no way to get the kids from daycare to school. The school suggested that we hire a taxi to pick up my daughter at daycare and drive her to school each day. As my oldest baby, this was not an option that I could stomach – hiring a stranger to pick up a 5 year old and drive her to and from daycare. Instead, we had her tested for intelligence to see if she would qualify for one of the schools in the area. Turns out the psychologist that tested her came back with a diagnosis of ADD. He said that when she found a task too difficult she would abandon it and this indicated ADD. Of course, the fact that she was only 4 meant that the diagnosis was not binding, according to him. We decided to enroll her and my son in a small private Lutheran School that was around the corner from our house. They enjoyed almost 2 years there. The challenge came in the second year when my daughter's struggles with reading became obvious. Unfortunately, the school was not prepared to diagnose, let alone implement, learning strategies to help her. We had to wait to find more pieces of the puzzle.

I joined the Junior League in Chicago and was mentioning some of our struggles with my daughter at a meeting. One of the women told me about her cousin who had been to the Pfeiffer Institute in Naperville. They took fecal, urine, hair and blood samples to put together compounded supplements designed for their patients. Right before we moved to the Dallas/Fort Worth area we took my daughter to this clinic. They suggested strict dietary changes and supplements. True to their prediction, she got worse before she got better. But better she did get...for a time.

When we made it to D/FW my daughter again struggled. At this point the first grade teacher said she didn't know how she made it out of Kindergarten because she couldn't read. We paid

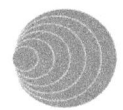

for her tutoring throughout the summer before second grade. Second grade came and yet again, we were told that she was not ready to advance. The entire summer of tutoring seemed to have been without effect. Somehow her teacher made it work for her in the classroom. We continued to work with her at home.

To even out the dynamics in the house we signed my son up for Kumon to give him "homework" when we were working with my daughter. This was a great thing. He had been learning to feign struggling so that he didn't have to complete activities he didn't feel like doing. He would get away with doing no work... Kumon helped him learn how to struggle and persevere. This also lightened our load as parents and allowed our daughter to get the one-on-one attention that she needed to progress with her reading.

Additionally, each of my children had Scouts. Focusing on non-academic activities allowed each of them to reach the levels that were comfortable for them without getting caught up with academic grades. I am so proud to say that I am the parent of a Gold Award Girl Scout and an Eagle Scout. The lesson here is to try different outlets for children until they find a spot where they can thrive and have success in at least one area of their life while they work on the others.

Another activity I encouraged my children to pursue was creative thinking. We would do "mommy homework" in the summer. I would pack a three-ringed binder with coloring pages, poems, simple word puzzles, anything that would be outside the standard school thinking. It was not a required activity, but when the boredom monster came out, so did the binder. It was a great success. Both kids also participated in Odyssey of the Mind and Destination Imagination. We only participated a couple of years, but the lessons of using the resources around you for solving the problems you are presented with have proven the test of time.

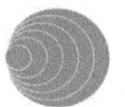

I had always wanted to teach my children German, but when my daughter's learning issues became apparent my husband asked me to let the German language school go and focus on the main schooling to not overload or depress our daughter. To continue the exposure to other cultures, we accepted an exchange student into our home at this time. We thought it would be a great fit. She had been around a small boy and had grown up on a farm in Germany. Turns out she couldn't stand being sniffed on by our dogs and she made a great fuss when my son was acting like a little boy at the dinner table. She lasted six months and then went to live with a house full of other teenagers. One never knows until trying what might work out or not, now we knew a little more about what to look for and what to say we would be offering.

Third grade rolled around for our daughter. We got another exchange student to see if we could have a better experience. This girl had also grown up on a farm. She had a little brother about the same age as our little guy. She fit in much better. In the end, she was with us for 11 months. We still communicate with her frequently.

This was the year that my daughter really started struggling. The third day of school she came home and sat in front of the TV and declared that she didn't care if she was able to watch TV or play with any of her friends, but she was not going to do any more homework or anything. I went to the school to raise the alarm. What I met with was an explanation from them that it was a parenting issue. I had a reclusive daughter and I needed to put her on medication for ADD, same as we had heard when she was four.

I was not convinced. None of her behaviors was consistent. We looked for additional information by getting our own psycho-educational evaluation. Basically, a second opinion. We were hoping for any kind of diagnosis to get some support from the school. Our own evaluation showed that our daughter was

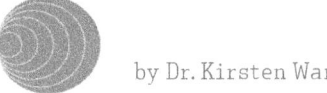

suffering with depression. We looked at the June Shelton School for Learning Differences in Dallas. They had specific tracks for students depending on their learning challenges. As a requirement for entry, any kind of mental challenge needed to be taken care of. We went to someone on their recommended list of therapists. This one man sent us to a psychiatrist to put her on medication. The psychiatrist informed us that since there was depression in the mix, the ADD could not be verified. She told us that depression poses many different symptoms that make any other diagnoses invalid until that first challenge could be resolved. We trusted her judgment and did not go the ADD medication route.

At the same time, the therapist told us that the dietary changes we had implemented were not effective and were ridiculous. My daughter was in the room when he said this and heard it. Now all bets were off. She ate whatever she wanted, whenever she wanted. While I knew this day would come, I didn't expect it this soon. When we went back to the psychiatrist I mentioned to her that I didn't see how we were going to be able to see if the medications she had given my daughter were working if all the rest of the lifestyle variables were not consistent. Lo and behold, the next time we went to the therapist he admitted that his giving nutritional advice was like him giving us advice about the cosmos and he knew really nothing about it. *Great.* I was the one dealing with an out of control 8 year old and he had washed his hands of the entire scenario. We felt bound to continue working with this therapist because of the Shelton requirements. Once our daughter had completed her on-site visit we were convinced that Shelton was a perfect fit for her – and so was she. The second day she returned from the visit she asked me, "Why doesn't my other school help me like this school does?" Of course, I didn't have any answers for that. The lesson from that is similar – keep researching and looking for that fit be it a therapist, school, diet or exercise program.

On my own health front, there were a lot of things going on. I found a new doctor and he put me on thyroid replacement therapy and other supplements. He added an occasional regime of B12 shots for energy. As is frequently seen, after a few months of feeling great on the thyroid medication the benefits wore off. I did not want to go on any stronger hormone replacement therapies. I needed to find something else. The hunt was on. I was optimistic because I had seen and felt benefits from the first regime, so I knew my body could get back to proper functioning somehow, if given the right supporting raw materials.

To help my daughter out with our eating restrictions, we had begun to make goodie bags for all her friends. In this way, even though she was not able to enjoy the cookies and candy that her friends did, she was able to hand out little trinkets to them instead. She really enjoyed being the center of attention in such a positive way.

She spent 5 years at Shelton. It was a great place for her. There was never any mention of ADD from them, and her depression lifted. The only treatments she was on during her time with them were nutritional supplements for her digestive tract issues, occupational therapy for her sensory integration dysfunction and dietary restrictions for her food sensitivities. She was beginning to mend. When she entered 4th grade we added chelation therapy to her treatment. She completed about 6 months and we were told by her teacher that she was making great strides in stamina during school. This stamina translated into an ability to deal with other students in a more positive manner. She was no longer getting irritated and overreacting about small events. She was continuing to mend.

I started looking at alternatives for work. When we got to D/FW I was trying to be a representative for the tool steel company. No one had covered the territory for ten years and this was a

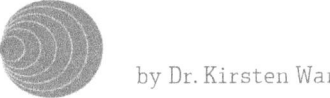
dying industry. I also found working out of the home challenging. In 2005 I decided to run the Dallas Marathon and then go back to school. With all that I had learned about health from my daughter, I thought that I would really like to do whole body healing. I looked at the Naturopathic route. My husband was not convinced. The school was far away and I had little kids. Wouldn't it be better to look for something that would fit into our current lifestyle? I went the pre-med route instead. Fitting classes in wherever I could, I went to several local universities and colleges to get the courses that would fit into my mommy schedule.

After a full two semesters in school we decided to move closer to Shelton because the commute was getting to be too much for our daughter. It was one hour each way, at a minimum. I had to take a break from school while we were getting the one house ready to sell and the other ready to move in. I would take the kids to school, pack up the dogs and go to the new house. There I would paint and do other kinds of sweaty labor until it was time to go back to pick up the kids again.

We moved to Far North Dallas after spring break. It was a good move. Both of my kids could ride their bicycles to school. Girl and Boy Scouts took up most of the weekends. Each one had an environment that was unique to them and they thrived.

My First Thermogram

When we got to North Dallas I found someone to help with my own health and get me off the thyroid supplements. The first step was to have a thermogram. My thermogram gave us a blueprint of what direction to take my care in. The thyroid was not my only problem. Turns out I had an acid/alkaline

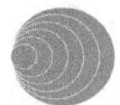

imbalance throughout my entire GI tract. Additionally, I had cystic fibrous breast tissue which was difficult to deal with during PMS times. My blood pressure was very low and needed support. One time when I was trying to give blood they measured 60/80 and asked me if I was still alive. Extreme dietary changes along with some very targeted therapies helped out.

Back to the Family Story

I discovered P90X at this time also. (A home exercise program developed by Tony Horton designed to take 90 days and combined with an eating plan.) It was wonderful. My body always loved the lactic acid build up. My weight still yo-yoed. Then I found HC3. (A homeopathic formula using the HcG hormone produced by the body during pregnancy to metabolize fat as an energy source for the baby.) That worked like a charm but threw my hormones off balance. Not only were my hormones off, but increased stress threw my entire system off again. Good health is a continual process, remember it not only changes as we age, but changed in response to the environment we live in.

After 8th grade my daughter wanted to go back to public school. She attended the local high school. I decided to check out the local community college for my son to go to so that he could receive the challenges that he needed. At the orientation meeting, my daughter fell in love with the school. She decided that she wanted to make the switch for 11th and 12th grade. And this from a kid that Shelton said would not survive in public school. She graduated from Richland Collegiate High School with an associate's degree. Her college was completed in 2.5 years and she is now on her own, in a city of her own choosing and enjoying her new freedom.

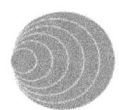

My son took the more conventional route and finished high school with numerous AP credits. He is at The University of Texas and earned the president's scholarship.

My husband and I have downsized and are ready to continue our lives with a slower pace and hope that we can help others with the journey to better health and wellness.

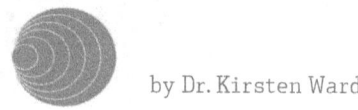

Chapter Six:
How to Evaluate YOUR Body

So now you have seen some of the ups and downs I went through with my health and the health of my children. The key was to always keep assessing my body and how the treatments I was trying were affecting me – good, bad AND mixed results!

Reasons for our body not having the right nutrients:

Of course, we all know that eating only fast foods or other junk foods just won't have in them some of the things our body needs. In fact, obese people can actually be malnourished! This is an easy issue to understand and to start to fix. BUT, this is NOT THE WHOLE STORY.

Sometimes the veggies we eat have been grown in soil that is not healthy – not rich in nutrients. Therefore, that lovely tomato may be little more than water and fiber.

Sometimes our own digestive tract may not be working efficiently, so even if the input of food is sufficient in quality and nutrients, our bodies are not pulling all the needed materials from that food and it just passes through our system.

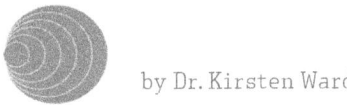

These are the 3 top reason that our internal organs, well, even our skin, may not be functioning at their very best.

- Junk Food
- Poor Quality Food
- Your Own Digestive System

Solution

So what is a person to do? Let's take them in order. Junk food is the easiest – cut it out. Each person must decide if they can tolerate it in any amount, and remember – what you could put down (eat) and feel healthy with when you were 18 is vastly different than what you can put down and feel healthy with at 40! So maybe your favorite ice cream or candy bar is now just a treat on your birthday instead of a weekly routine. There are always those few people with a great metabolism who can eat what they want at any time and in any amount. Realize you have to evaluate YOUR body and not compare this to what others eat. Besides, do you really know the digestive problems they may have? The behavior and mood issues they may struggle with? You don't know the whole story just by seeing what they are eating. So cut out the junk food and the fast food as a routine part of your eating and add some back in if you must – evaluating how little bits make you feel when stretched out over time.

Next is the quality of food you are eating. Some people are very sensitive to pesticides, some are not. Some people are very sensitive to fibers and probiotics and so on ... again this goes back to the empowerment issue – try things, evaluate and eliminate or add according to what results you get. Keep an eating diary and record how you feel minutes to hours after eating certain items.

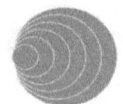

For some people, spending on organic food is not worth the cost. For some it is necessary. However let me add a little known and very important part of this issue – organic plants have longer roots on average. *Hum? What does that have to do with things?* Well, the deeper the roots go down in soil that is organic (no pesticides, fungicides and other stuff) the more pure minerals and other nutrients those roots pick up. Soil with chemicals used on it kills the earthworms and the good fungi, so they stop living in it and mixing up the minerals – so it has to be living soil for this benefit to reach your food.

The more trace minerals that the roots pick up, the more will be found in your tomato! So there is another and little known aspect to choosing your food. I highly recommend going on an all organic food plan to start off and then if you must, add back in one item at a time and record in your journal or diary how that addition makes you feel. Give each addition a full week or two before adding any new item to make sure you are allowing the affect to fully be felt so you can eliminate it as a problem causer.

And lastly – your own digestive system! Whether your digestive track is not working well to start out – or deficiencies have slowed it down and now you are caught in a vicious cycle – you will need to take supplements and/or eat more of the foods that have what your body needs to ensure you get enough nutrients to allow your digestive system to begin to heal itself. As your body heals and changes, you can adjust, reduce and even eliminate some of these. The absorption of fats, carbohydrates, proteins, vitamins, minerals: all this will play a part in if, how fast, and when your digestive system gets back to normal. A simple potato "contains over a hundred and fifty known chemical substances and many unknown chemical substances as well." (Pederson 1994) Remember that fibers (soluble and insoluble) are as important as nutrients – providing a structure and also 'capturing' material as it passes through your system.

This is a lot to juggle – a lot to know. Don't Panic! Your health specialist will be working with you to draw up an eating and exercising plan and will gladly share with you ideas and knowledge about all of these areas. Often even a meditation/stress reduction portion will be added to your health plan. You will not be alone on this journey.

Here is a little nugget to showcase even further how complex our bodies are – and why you can't just evaluate once in your lifetime and run on those results ... Your body is constantly monitoring and balancing fluids, functions and actions with the building blocks that you provide for it. The choices you make on what you put into your body directly provides those available building blocks for the body to use. We really are what we eat. Our bodies cannot obtain building blocks from things that we do not make available to it. Water, food, fiber, exercise, outside temperature and humidity – my oh my! Just remember, once you have learned some of these things, they become as easy to think about as tying your shoes, so do NOT feel overwhelmed, you will have plenty of help along the way, plenty of guidance and input as you work on your plan and it gets easier and easier as you go along.

Having your baseline thermogram and then setting up a schedule for follow up thermograms will be one of your best tools in this journey back to optimal health. Remember that all this works in consort (connection) with your primary care doctor. This is an enhancement tool, not your only tool! The key is working to RESTORE your body to health.

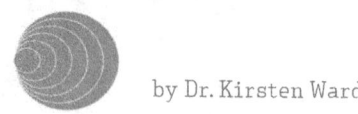

Chapter Seven:
Mammogram Controversy

I have to stress for legal reason, and because we aren't face to face allowing me to personalize any information: that all information in this book and especially this section is for informational purposes only and is not meant to give you individual medical advice. As mentioned many times earlier in this book, each person is different (physical, mental, genetic, environmental) and therefore all care plans must be carried out after an in-person consultation. The information here is GENERAL information meant to help educate you – to empower you in taking a vital and energetic part in your own health care.

Do I or don't I have a mammogram this year?

What is the controversy and do I really have a choice?

These are questions I hear all the time. In the United States the mammogram has become the gold standard for breast health.

Why do other countries not follow this lead?

What do men and women do to monitor their breast and whole body health if not with mammograms?

We will take a tour of other methods for determining health and disease that people in other parts of the world use. Think

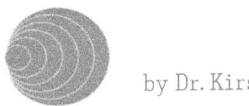

about how these might enhance the healing outlook for people here in our country.

When the United States revised the recommendations about mammogram screenings, there was mass confusion, frustration and disbelief from women who were convinced that the only way to find tumors in their breast tissue was through mammography. Explanations about why these revisions were made and what the alternatives were was not very well explained. Mostly people got a 20 second blurb about it on the nightly news!

Let's revisit the reasons for the revised recommendations and explore some of the alternatives.

Mammograms have been held up as the holy grail of breast health in our country. Yearly screenings used to be recommended for as long as I can remember. With a reevaluation of the data, some startling facts have come to light:

1. The small number of women who have actually been helped
2. Large number of women whose cancer was not found by Mammograms
3. Large number of women who had been diagnosed with a false positive who went through long and agonizing treatments and mental anguish

A word or two about infra-red camera thermography: The IR camera takes a snapshot of the hot and cold zones on a body. Not all tumors are hot and not all tumors are cold. This ONE snapshot is not able to indicate the numerous signature patterns that Whole Body Regulation Thermography can since it is coupled with its data base of thousands of documented cases. These signatures can add to the terrain picture by illuminating systemic viral infections, underlying heavy metals, a body's inability to detoxify efficiently, pH imbalances and food intolerances, among other things. This is

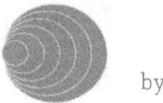

not to discount IR camera thermography, just a need to highlight and know the differences. (For more information read the book: *How Doctors Think*)

Citing from the above book: Mammography is routinely ordered by primary care physicians as a screening test to detect early cancer in women entering middle age. "Mammograms are the most monotonous type of work that we do," Orwig said. "And mammograms are the most anxiety provoking of all x-rays," he added. To miss a cancer is devastating, because the tumors that are found early are readily removed, and missing the cancer can result in metastases that are hard to control and rarely, if ever, cured. On the other hand, over reading a mammogram will subject a healthy woman to the emotional rollercoaster of further imaging, a biopsy and then the lingering doubt about whether there actually was a cancer that was missed despite the biopsy result. Not surprisingly, mammography is a fertile field for medical-legal conflict, and radiologists are acutely aware that errors can result in a malpractice lawsuit. Even the best radiologists will inaccurately read a mammogram in 2 to 3% of the cases, while some series show that other doctors incorrectly read the images in (page 187) 20% or more. The aim is to recommend a biopsy on the women who will prove to have a tumor, and not to recommend a biopsy for women with benign changes on their mammogram. The women who undergo a biopsy are said to be 'called back.' "In theory, it would be best to have a four or five percent callback rate," Orwig said. This is considered to be the optimal rate. "But the norm," Orwig said, "is about ten to eleven percent." This higher call back rate results in a larger number of women with benign changes who undergo further evaluation and biopsy.

There is a tradeoff here: causing emotional distress in women with benign changes versus the need to 'capture' a number of breast cancers that otherwise would be missed. In Orwig's group of 11 radiologists, he falls in the call back rate of 10%, the norm, but one colleague has a 16% call back rate. Many of

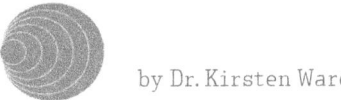

the women he calls back end up having benign biopsies. "He was sued," Orwig told me. "Years ago he missed a breast cancer." This experience caused him to become more 'aggressive,' as Orwig put it, in assessing mammograms and calling more women back for further studies and biopsy. While his colleague's call back rate is still within reasonable bounds, there is no doubt that the consequences of missing a malignant lesion and being sued caused him to think in a different way. Dr. Potchen published a paper analyzing medical decision-making and concluded that what most influenced clinical choices was "the last bad experience." Potchen's conclusion mirrors the availability error, which Croskerry and Redelmeir highlighted earlier: what is most available in your mind strongly colors your thinking about a new case that has some similarities, but it can cause you to ignore important differences and come to an incorrect diagnosis. (page 188)

Still citing *How Doctors Think*: Given the difficulties in perception and cognition that Kundel and other researchers have reported, could computers replace radiologists or at least lower their error rates? One computer-aided diagnostic system was approved in 2006 by the Food and Drug Administration for identifying lung nodules on chest x-rays. Other systems are being studied, including those for mammograms. The pivotal clinical trial on malignant lung nodules that led to the FDA approval involved 15 radiologists who were asked to note their level of suspicion that a chest x-ray contained cancer. They used a scoring system of 1 to 100, and they were to mark the location that caused their suspicion. Eighty cancer cases and 160 cancer-free cases were in the study. Each radiologist interpreted these 240 cases three times: two times separated by one to four months without computer assistance and then, immediately after the second interpretation, with computer assistance.

Computer assistance improved detection of the cancer between 14 and 24%, depending on its size. But the computer system also

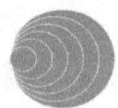

caused radiologists to change almost 10% of their correct decisions (identifying the cancer) to incorrect diagnoses (stating that it was unimportant or benign). Of the 15 radiologists in the clinical trial, no two had identical results in evaluating the 80 cancer cases and 160 cancer-free cases. All but 25% of the cancers were identified by all 15 radiologists. But the difficult-to-diagnose cancers were found by only 4 of the radiologists. No radiologist identified all 80 of the cancers correctly.

One unwelcome effect of computer-assisted detection was that after being prompted by the computer, more radiologists suspected cancer in chest x-rays that came from patients without a malignancy – a false-positive reading. This demonstrates the power of technology, particularly computer-based, in shaking the confidence of a specialist in their initial diagnosis. It also demonstrates that machines do not provide perfect solutions to the imperfection of perception and thinking. Perhaps, as radiologists become more accustomed to computer-assisted detection and receive clinical feedback about the risk of becoming overly suspicious about benign findings on a chest x-ray, they will accommodate their thinking to the new technology. In the meantime, as they search for another new middle ground, there will be a tradeoff, with more accurate cancer detection but greater patient anxiety, as more people without cancer are subjected to the emotional upheaval and invasive procedures that follow on false positives. (p. 199)

More: In screening mammography, a sample of 110 radiologists who interpreted the mammograms of 148 women, the fraction of patients actually having cancer who were correctly diagnosed varied from 59 to 100%, and the fraction of patients without disease who were correctly diagnosed as normal ranged from 35 to 98%. Overall, the accuracy rate varied from 73 to 97%. (p. 181) [End citation of *How Doctors Think*]

Other Direct Citations

- Regular mammogram screenings do not reduce breast cancer death rates according to the British Medical Journal (2014;348).
- Effective cancer screening methods are important, but mammography is simply NOT a safe or effective cancer screen. Instead, I strongly advise to consider the safer and more effective alternative of thermographic breast screening. (Dr. Joseph Mercola, DO; 7/28/2015)
- The Swiss Medical Board no longer recommends mammograms. (New England Journal of Medicine 2014: 270: 1965-1967
- Experts do not advise routine mammograms for women under 50. Despite numerous testimonials from women who believe "a mammogram saved my life," the truth is that most women who find breast cancer as a result of regular screening have not had their lives saved by the test, conclude two Dartmouth researchers, Dr. H. Gilbert Welch and Brittney A. Frankel ... Translated into real numbers, that means screening mammography helps 4,000 to 18,000 women each year. Although those numbers are not inconsequential, they represent just a small portion of the 230,000 women given a breast cancer diagnosis each year, and a fraction of the 39 million women who undergo mammograms each year in the United States. Dr. Welch says it's important to remember that of the 138,000 women found to have breast cancer each year as a result of mammography screening, 120,000 to 134,000 are not helped by the test ... Of all the women who have a screening test who have breast cancer detected, and eventually survive the cancer, the vast majority would have survived anyway. Dr. Begg said, "It only saved the lives of a very small fraction of them."

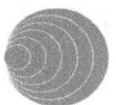

(https://well.blogs.nytimes.com/201110/24/mammogram s-role-as-savor-is-tested/?emc=eta1&_r=1)

- Research from the longest and largest study on mammograms shows mammograms are NOT beneficial. Here is a quote: "It [study] found that the death rates from breast cancer and from all causes were the same in women who got mammograms and those who did not. And the screening had harms: One in five cancers found with mammography and treated was not a threat to the woman's health and did not need treatment such as chemotherapy, surgery or radiation ... Dr. Peter Juni, a member of the Swiss Medical Board until recently, said one concern was that mammography was not reducing the overall death rate from the disease, but increasing over diagnosis and leading to false positives and needless biopsies ... Dr. Kalager compared mammography to prostate-specific antigen screening for prostate cancer, using data from pooled analyses of clinical trials. It turned out that the two screening tests were almost identical in their over diagnosis rate and had almost the same slight reduction in breast or prostate deaths." (https://www.nytimes.com/2014/02/12/health/study-adds-new-doubts-about-value-of-mammograms.html?_r=0)

- "In addition to early detection and accurate test results, here are some other reasons I like thermography: 1. Good for young, dense breasts and implants; 2. Detect cell changes in the arm pit area; 3. Great additional test (can be used as an additional test to help...make more informed...decisions); 4. It doesn't hurt; 5. No radiation; 6. Thermography is very safe ... In honor of Breast Health Awareness Month, I encourage you to check out thermography for yourself and your loved ones!" Christiane Northrup, MD https://www.facebook.com/DrChristianeNorthrup. *The Best Breast Cancer Screening Tests.* Christiane Northrup MD. Oct. 2016.

- "The use of medical imaging with high-dose radiation – CT scans in particular – has soared in the last 20 years. Our resulting exposure to medical radiation has increased more than six fold between the 1980s and 2006, according to the National Council on Radiation Protection & Measurements. The radiation doses of CT scans (a series of x-ray images from multiple angles) are 100 to 1,000 times higher than conventional x-rays ... The relationship between radiation and the development of cancer is well understood: A single CT scan exposes a patient to the amount of radiation that epidemiologic evidence shows can be cancer causing ... CTs, once rare, are now routine. One in 10 Americans undergo a CT scan every year, and many of them get more than one." https://www.nytimes.com/2014/01/31/opinion/we-are-giving-ourselves-cancer.html

- "Thermography is predominantly a risk marker for breast pathology procedure which is non-invasive and non-compressive. Perhaps the most pertinent evidence comes from an extensive cohort study of 58,000 patients over a 12 year span that made a significant contribution to the evaluation of patients suspected of having breast cancer ... Therefore as soon as a suspicious (positive) breast thermal examination is performed, the appropriate follow-up diagnostic and clinical testing can be ordered. This would include mammography and other imaging tests, clinical laboratory procedures, nutritional and lifestyle evaluation and training in breast self examination. Thermography is a simple, non-invasive, highly accurate, inexpensive form of diagnostic imaging as well as a "breast friendly" procedure. ... in a healthy individual, body temperature is kept constant in a very small range despite large differences in temperature of the surroundings and also those in physical activity. Strict regulation of body temperature, necessary for optimal progress of

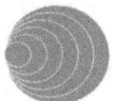

enzymatic reactions, is developed in all homoitermic animals that include humans."
https://www.academia.edu/7514453/Contact-Thermography_a_scientific_evaluation

That is a wide range of information all from well-developed nations and their scientists. These studies don't say never have a mammogram; they do recommend other ways to go about when and why to have one than most U.S. woman are used to.

Will Thermography Diagnose Cancer

No! Please realize thermography is a functional test, so it shows the functioning of your organs. If a tumor is preventing the optimal functioning of your organ, it will show up as an organ that is struggling with its function. The test itself does not necessarily show a diagnosis at any point, but it does show weakness in the functioning of the organs. That would indicate possible areas for future testing, depending on how compromised those functions are. This is all in line with the scientific research cited above. So if you feel a lump, certainly have it checked out with a thermogram and decide with your doctor if you need further tests.

CASE STUDY #5

Person #5 is a 45 year old woman who came for a thermogram because she was having a bloody discharge from her right breast. Her mammography showed microcalcifications and her biopsy was negative but guarded with a lumpectomy recommended.

Person #5's report highlighted six main areas of concern, which then became the priority areas for treatment plans. Her lymph system was blocked, she had extreme temperature difference from one breast to the other, she had indications of myocardium danger and food sensitivity as well as indications of toxins in her body.

A CBC blood test was ordered, as well as probiotic therapy and lymph supporting supplements. Heart supplements were also added and food sensitivities were tested and she was on a diet elimination plan. The results also connected to dental issues and she had root canals removed, then went through both a liver and a brain detox program.

At the initial testing, Person #5 was positive for 8 out of 12 suspicion criteria (your practitioner will explain these at your first visit) and after her treatment plans she was at 2 out of 12 suspicion criteria with no other treatment but those recommended from her thermogram results.

Breast Cancer in Particular

I am often asked if I can do just a breast thermogram. A Whole Body Thermogram gives you an indication of how the body as a whole functions as a unit. Since you don't go through life just as a hand, having just a hand scan is not as valuable as having the whole body scanned, especially if whatever is growing on the hand didn't originate in the hand. So we only offer whole body thermogram because everything is interrelated in the human body.

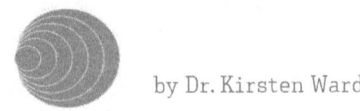

Chapter Eight:
History to CSI Episodes

This is a fun chapter, we start with a mud bath and go all the way to a hit TV show. All this to establish a very long and successful history in using thermal bio-scanning as a way to assess the health of the human body.

Way back in 480 BC (that's about 2,500 years ago) the father of caring medicine, Hippocrates, used mud on his patients to find areas that would dry first – those areas would give him an indication of which internal organs were working harder than they were supposed to. Of course, the treatment course taken after diagnosis back then lacks the finesse we offer today! No lizard toe tea for us now.

When the scientific method, operated under logical observation, started to become the norm, the WHY of the issue of hot body spots was looked into. Claude Bernard (1813-1878) studied this and described how our bodies attempt to maintain a very steady level of heat. He also found our bodies work to have that same even level in hydration (water). Keeping the core (inside) of our bodies at a very even and steady temperature is what our organ systems need in order for the enzymes to make their work possible. Enzyme shape is very VERY temperature sensitive. It really is true that just a few degrees hotter will indicate trouble.

A generation after this, R. N. Lawson did work related to cancer. He discovered that the skin temperature over a cancer area was higher than other normal skin areas. In 1956 he showed the venous blood draining from the tumor site was often warmer than the arterial blood supply going into the tumor site.

At the same time Lawson was starting his studies in Canada, the dental connection to health was being studied by Weston Price and Dr. Arno Rost. Over 50 disease signatures were found and substantiated using data from thousands of patients over a 15 year study period.

In the late 1970s and early 1980s another push about diagnosis of disease and the body's ability to regulate temperature was underway. Alfred Pischinger, Hans Seyle and others were busy putting together more pieces of the puzzle and started using the term thermography. This work lead to the investigation by the FDA which then lead to thermography being cleared as an Adjunct Diagnosis tool in 1997 – listed out especially for:

- Abnormalities of the female breast
- Peripheral vascular disease
- Musculosketal disorders
- Extracranial cerebral and facial vascular disease
- Abnormalities of the thyroid gland
- Various neoplastic and inflammatory conditions

And as a newly approved FDA procedure, a computer program was developed to make the reading of thermograms free from human error by using computers to crunch the result numbers. This takes us right up to modern times ...

... Where we find developments in machines and theories have put thermography in the forefront of many sciences – including forensic science. On the hit TV show, CSI, you will see the officers using various tools to process the scene of a crime and gather evidence and clues. Temperature differation is even being tested to replace luminol!

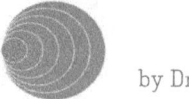

The U.S. government has been using thermal images for search and rescue missions, fugitive recovery and other uses for decades. In Europe they have been using thermography for over 50 years, it was cleared by their health care systems many years before being cleared by the U.S. FDA. So this type of diagnosis tool has a *very long* and *Very Safe* history.

The beauty of what you get from your thermogram results is that they are all shared with your doctor and then you have the information in your hand – empowering you to address the systems in your body potentially 8-10 years before those systems finally breakdown ... You're being given the opportunity to fix things about you ten years before they show up as a structural change. So you have a golden opportunity to make changes in your life. But it's up to you and your doctor as to what you want to do with it. Again, empower yourself and learn about the areas your thermogram says are working too hard – are working abnormally – are working too sluggishly - and these warnings signs indicate they will be breaking down in the future if not given the materials and environment they need to heal themselves.

A thermogram is a really good basic procedure that tells you how your body is functioning as a whole. If you are an individual who is interested in feeling better and living a long life that's full of activity and ... free from pain and discomfort ... a thermogram is in your best interest. You will see things on there that show you the areas your body is struggling with which you may not have known about or felt any discomfort about yet.

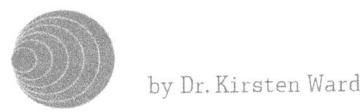

Chapter Nine:
LISTEN TO YOUR BODY

Western and allopathic medicine is first rate in the "acute care model." We certainly do not want to replace any medical care, emergency care or other medical attention you receive from you doctors for things like emergency pain, car accidents, other accident and such other types of immediate needs.

However, it does not fare so well with chronic problems that can be "caused or worsened by our lifestyle choices" (*A Thyme to Heal*). If a diagnostic tool as sensitive as those used in thermography offers the ability to get to the root of the causes before the symptoms become unmanageable for the individual, then a person is offered many other avenues to help in healing, while also offering an opportunity to monitor progress.

Human nature is to only focus on problems, therefore as you learn and feel empowered about your choices, the one guiding light you need to keep in mind is to listen when your body gives you clues.

Modern life is busy! We have to go to work, we have to keep up with children, clubs, meetings, shopping, schooling ... it really is a packed scheduled that we all have. Certainly it is much more time efficient if you have a slightly pulled muscle, or an odd little rumble in your tummy to just power through that small body dysfunction and keep on keeping on ... hum?

Or is it?

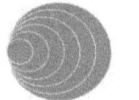

If you know you reached too far (sports or cleaning the house or whatever) and pulled a muscle, and it is sore the next day – then you have listened to your body, and you know what caused that sore feeling. Under normal circumstances, all you have to do is not over use that muscle for a few days and you will back to normal. That is reasonable.

BUT ...

If you have a sore muscle and you don't recall a physical pull or over use as the reason, pay attention; monitor it. If it stays sore for days – getting worse or even staying the same – then your body is giving you a clue that something inside is not functioning as it should be. This gives you TIME to figure out what is going wrong and start to treat it before it breaks down and affects more muscles or your breathing or becomes a very dangerous life-threatening condition.

The tummy ... if you have a rumble in your tummy and you know you ate too much, certainly have some mint or ginger and let your body work on the extra digestion. If you don't recall anything as a reasonable cause, then your body is giving you a clue that something is not functioning as it should be!

Don't be like my parents who waited until I was routinely throwing up my morning juice to look at the problem and change things – I was lucky I did not have permanent digestive damage, perhaps because I was so young at the time and my body was still developing – so that the offending food was taken away in time for my internal organs to heal themselves.

Are you picking up the pattern here? You must listen to your body when it is quietly giving you clues that things are just not okay – if you don't – then you will be dealing with very serious and costly medical care while your body is screaming and throwing a tantrum to finally get your attention and fix it before a major breakdown.

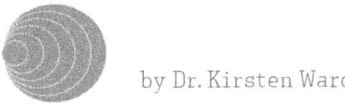

A book like this cannot list out every type of clue your body may be giving you – remember we are all different – so the parameters are for you to know your body. How does it feel when you are thinking you feel at your best? How does it feel when you know you overate a little? How does it feel when you pull a muscle or twist an ankle?

THEN ... take that knowledge and if you aren't feeling your best for a while, if your tummy is feeling oddly, if that muscle pull is not really the same exact pain as a 'normal' sore muscle – then you really need to address these issues before they get worse.

Please realize I am NOT telling you wait to have a thermogram until you are picking up clues from your body that something is not right. I suggested earlier that you get a baseline thermogram and then have one at every yearly checkup – they are not expensive and from going into the treatment center to going out – they take up very little time – about an hour. However, if you haven't had a thermogram yet and you realize you are now getting warning clues from your body; now is the time to not put it off anymore and get that thermogram!

We have looked at how the body ideally utilizes carbohydrates, fats and proteins as well as the micronutrients of vitamins and minerals and enzymes. When the balance of these elements is thrown off by disease or lifestyle choice, the body attempts to regain balance. In the process of regaining balance the body displays certain 'symptoms' that allopathic medicine attempts to control and suppress. Don't treat the symptoms, treat the cause and the symptoms will go away once good health is restored.

Natural health practitioners aim to look for the root causes of the symptoms and provide your body the necessary supports to help it heal itself. I have seen great success using thermograms as a diagnostic tool for finding root causes and have also seen many poorly functioning digestive tracts as a major struggle for those individuals who are ailing. I have seen these people work back to a healthy and pain free life after working with me on a treatment plan. Therefore, the first place to support healing in an ailing individual is usually to heal the digestive tract. A normally functioning digestive tract enables the body to obtain the necessary nutrients which we discussed are so very important for all our internal systems.

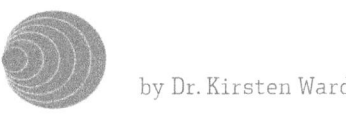
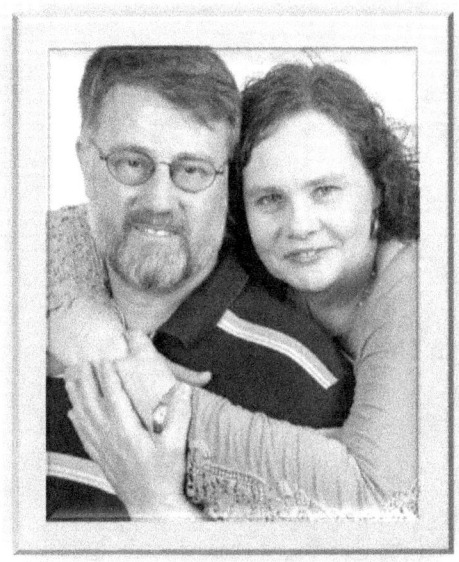

About The Author

Kirsten is a Naturopathic Doctor and President & Founder of Ridglea Wellness. When Kirsten is not helping people with naturopathic healing she has many varied interests. Kirsten has taught high school Biology, Chemistry and Physics.

Kirsten raised a husband, two kids and multiple critters that include dogs, cats, toads, fish, bearded dragons and a boa snake. Most of her non-human family has been acquired from rescue shelters.

At an early age, Kirsten developed a love for fiber arts from her grandmother. She eventually learned to needlepoint, cross-stitch, knit, weave, spin and dye yarn. If you ever see her wearing something knitted - it was probably homemade. Vacations are centered around visiting yarn stores and farms where she can meet the animals (alpaca or sheep) and buy fleece to be turned into a one of a kind creation. Recently Kirsten helped introduce the Knitted Knockers in Fort Worth to offer soft knit prosthetics for cancer survivors.

Kirsten has a deep love of the outdoors. In high school she completed a 64 day training course at Hurricane Island. She then joined the Wilderness Skills club at Vanderbilt and enjoyed hiking, camping & backpacking with family in Tennessee, Oklahoma, Texas, New York, Maine, Vermont, New Mexico & Colorado. She has even summited Guadalupe Mountain and Wheeler Peak the highest points in TX & NM. Kirsten's love of the outdoors got her involved with the Boy Scouts of America, taking on adult leadership roles in Cub Scouts, Boy Scouts and Venturing.

After all the above Kirsten also found time to volunteer with the Junior League of Chicago, Fort Worth and Dallas. Plus, she has socialized dogs at Operation Kindness, delivered meals for Meals on Wheels and served as a Gold Award Councilor with the Girl Scouts of Northeast Texas.

Please contact Kirsten at: website: www.ridgleawellness.com and the email: info@ridgleawellness.com

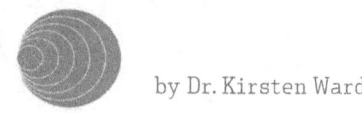

Appendix One

Using Food to Influence the Body in Growth, Maintenance and
Repair

Kirsten Irmtraud Lorenz Ward

August 18, 2017

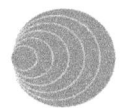

Upon completion of a medical school degree newly graduated medical doctors pledge what many people know as the Hippocratic Oath (Hulkower, 2016, p. 42). The staying power of this oath is that "it represents one's commitment to the Hippocratic tradition – a tradition based upon sound scientific investigation combined with patient-oriented care." (Hulkower, 2016, p. 43) While the Oath has mistakenly been shortened to "do no harm," the actual text is much more nuanced. It is widely available to read in its entirety, but the part that is of interest to us reads: "there is art to medicine as well as science, and that warmth, sympathy, and understanding may outweigh the surgeon's knife or the chemist's drug." (Librarian, n.d.) It is this part of the oath that seems to be overlooked today. Recently, a 74 year-old woman in Florida hired a Concierge Doctor to whom she paid a retainer fee for guaranteed access to services. Finding herself feeling under the weather, she decided to go to the doctor. This happened to be a day when the doctor was not in the office. Instead of having an actual visit with the woman, the office called in a prescription to the pharmacy for antibiotics and steroids. This encounter runs in direct opposition to the oath that clearly states "warmth, sympathy, and understanding…outweigh…the chemist's drug." It is for this reason that I have pursued a degree from Trinity School of Natural Health. As Dr. Vogel so eloquently phrased it: "Today's orthodox medical opinion in the main still holds to the fundamentally wrong view that it is the illness or disease itself, the symptom, that has to be treated and if possible combatted or suppressed by strong drugs." (Vogel & Selbert, 1991, Preface) Restoring health is the goal of all medical practitioners. The methods of achieving this goal differ from tradition to tradition, but: "If we want to live healthy, happy and joyful lives, we must endeavor to reestablish the proper relationship between ourselves – the whole body and mind – and nature." (Vogel & Selbert, 1991, Preface) The body is always in a state of flux and change with the goal of maintaining a desired equilibrium; otherwise known as homeostasis. When we look at a body trying to heal and readjust itself, what we see as "symptoms" are not necessarily something that

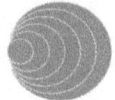

need fixing or repairing. Time and the body's own natural healing systems will take care of itself if given the proper support.

So how can we find what the root causes are of the symptoms that we observe? The objective observation and testing of individuals is very important. When "the traditional targets – blood and urine (and sometimes hair) - do not always give the most useful information" (Biesalski & Tinz, 2017, p. 77), then something different is needed. Trinity teaches the Reams' Biological Theory of Ionization (RBTI) and I look forward to trying that diagnostic tool, but I have years of experience working with Whole Body Regulation Thermography and Thermometry. This is a non-invasive testing tool that uses a hand-held thermometer-sensor with a germanium crystal that filters infra-red photons at precise points located on the dermatomes of the body. These dermatomes are controlled by single nerves from the spinal cord. These nerves, in turn, are related to the specific organ or organ system that is found directly beneath them ("Spinal Nerves Up Close - SpinalHub," n.d.). They are similar to Traditional Chinese Medicine body meridians.

After initial readings are taken with the subject in a comfortably warm environment, the subject is then exposed to a light environmental stressor – cooling in a tightly controlled environment (68-73° F) in which the subject remains standing and disrobed for ten minutes. This light stressor should result in the body responding with a viscero-cutaneous reflex arc. ("Principles of Manual Medicine: Reflex Activity," n.d.) Ideally this means that the blood is restricted to the area that is most important for survival: the body core and brain after the stress. A new set of measurements is then taken. With the data collected through these measurements, a highly sophisticated mathematical algorithm calculates specific "signature patterns" that are identified and verified with over 30 years of clinical research including blood tests, other imaging types and biopsies. (Rost, 1985, pp. 22–24) This part of the evaluation is called Thermometry. It removes human subjectivity errors in the calculations and presents the top six imbalances as compared to over

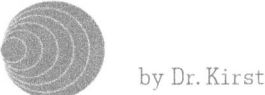

40 different disease types and dysfunctions. (Family and Environmental Medicine, 2015). The sensitivity of the test allows for dysfunction to be observed up to 8-10 years before structural changes in the tissues are visible (Liesha Getson, 2016). Whole Body Thermography and Thermometry are an extremely powerful tool in determining the actual functioning of body systems. Targeted preventative measures can then be decided upon to address these dysfunctions before structural changes become harder to correct. "Too much of so-called natural courses of treatment can also lead to excessive regulation, which demands an immediate slowing down of therapeutic efforts. One notices that there are remarkably sensitive patients who cannot be treated carefully enough. Again the thermogram helps."(Rost & Rost, 1990, p. 77) Basically, follow up thermograms can determine the efficacy of these treatments at the sub-clinical level.

According to Lutz and Mazzur, disease can be prevented "on three levels: primary, secondary and tertiary." (Lutz, 2015) At the primary prevention level the goal is to "avert the occurrence of disease." The secondary prevention level is designed to utilize "monitoring techniques to discover incipient diseases early enough to enhance the opportunity to control their effects." The tertiary prevention level is where nutrition is used as a treatment "after a disease has occurred to prevent complications or to promote maximum adaptation." The common thread at every one of these levels of prevention is the application of principles of nutrition that optimize individual body healing.

Through years of experience with Whole Body Thermography, I have witnessed that most individuals complaining of a variety of ailments present with the signatures patterns related to physiological compensation (acid and alkaline imbalance), food intolerance, food sensitivity, dysbiosis (mycosis or bacterial infection) and putrification (Beilin, p. 19). These dysfunctions are all directly related to a badly functioning gastrointestinal tract. To promote healing in a body with these types of dysfunction, it is of utmost importance to heal the digestive tract first. The digestive tract lays the ground work for the body to heal itself. Without the proper building blocks repair is challenging, if not impossible. "National health care expenditures for 1990 totaled $666 billion of which 30% are related to inappropriate diet." (Bidlack, 1996)

For growth, maintenance and repair, the body uses ingested items both as sources of energy and as nutrients for necessary functioning. In other words: ingested food is used by the body as building blocks. Those building blocks can be used as energy in the form of calories or as raw materials for repair and replacement. With bodies that already possess a compromised digestive tract, it becomes even more crucial to optimize the nutritional components and energy resources from the ingested nutrients.

To date it has been discovered that the body requires approximately 50 essential factors that must come from our environment. These include: 20 or 21 minerals, 13 vitamins, 9 essential amino acids, 2 essential fatty acids, water, oxygen, light and a source of energy (usually starch or glucose). (Erasmus, 1993, p. 6) Drinking lots of good quality water, consuming high quality foods with dense nutrients, exposing the skin to sunlight in a healthy way and breathing lots of clean air, is the best way to achieve a good quality of life. Living in today's world most of the individuals I have crossed paths with have presented with compromised digestive tracts that negatively impact the goal of having a good quality of life. This paper will discuss the various ways in which food substances are an integral part of the healing required in individuals with compromised digestive tracts. We will look at how to optimize the bioavailability of ingested items for the dysfunctioning population and thereby support individual healing. We will start by looking at how the ideally functioning body utilizes the various components.

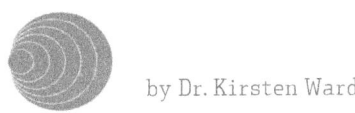

How normal digestion and absorption should occur

A normally functioning gastrointestinal tract processes carbohydrates, fats and proteins (amino acids linked by peptide linkages/bonds) in order to break them down into absorbable components that are then used by the body to live, maintain and grow. The other micronutrients (vitamins and minerals) are processed differently and will be discussed later.

Digestion in the Mouth

Upon entry into the human body all ingested items are broken down mechanically by the teeth and chemically by the digestive enzyme ptyalin (an αamylase). This enzyme is secreted by glands located in the back of the mouth. Only carbohydrates are responsive to the enzyme amylase (ideally pH 6.4). In the mouth proteins and fats are primarily being mechanically broken down by the teeth. It must be noted that a small portion of triglycerides (one kind of ingested fat) become digested with the aid of the lingual lipase secretion from the lingual glands. These glands are located at the back of the tongue, near the taste buds. Water as a crucial element in the body is introduced right at the beginning of digestion. All three, carbohydrates, proteins and fats, are being mixed with water from the saliva.

Since food only remains in the mouth for a short time, the digestion of carbohydrates is very brief. The entire mass now enters the stomach which has a vastly different environment from that of the mouth. Once in the stomach the pH is much lower than the pH in the mouth. This lower pH results in the inactivity of the amylase enzyme through denaturing. Denaturing is the external influence on a protein that changes the 3-Dimensional construction which can in turn affect the functioning of the molecule. The external forces required to cause an amino acid to denature are small and therefore require a tight range of pH levels to work.

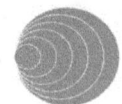

Hydrochloric acid, at a pH of around 0.8, is secreted by parietal cells in the stomach. The contracting and relaxing of the smooth muscle (peristalsis) that surrounds the stomach, continues the mechanical digestion. Once the food gets mixed in with the hydrochloric acid the pH in the stomach rises to a 2.0-3.0. This is the ideal environment for digestion within the stomach. Pepsin is the enzyme found in the stomach which digests the protein called collagen. This collagen is found primarily in the intercellular connective tissue of meats. Pepsin begins the process of breaking down the protein peptide linkages between the amino acids. About 10% of digested fat (in the form of triglycerides) is digested by the stomach with the aid of the mouth secretion lingual lipase. The stomach is not a good organ for absorption because it lacks villi for increased surface area, and absorptive epithelial cells. Only a very few highly fat soluble substances (alcohol and some drugs like aspirin) can be absorbed in small quantities in the stomach. (Hall & Guyton, 2011, p. 841) At this point the mass going through the digestive tract is called chyme and most of the heavy duty break down (digestion) begins.

Normal digestion in the small intestines

The small intestines are split into different parts, each of which has a specific name and function: duodenum, jejunum, ilium. The duodenum is the upper portion of the small intestines. The jejunum is in the middle and the ilium is the latter. The duodenum and upper jejunum are where the bulk of the digestion takes place. In addition to mechanical digestion, peristalsis in the small intestines has the added task of encouraging the chyme to move down the entire length. The duodenum and upper jejunum is where the pancreas contributes large quantities of secretions of αamylase. In contrast to salivary amylase, the pancreatic secretions are more powerful. After 15-30 minutes of peristalsis almost all the carbohydrates will have been separated into maltose or other small glucose molecules. This same portion of the duodenum and upper jejunum is where proteins are digested with the help of the pancreatic secretions collectively known as proleotytic enzymes (individually: trypsin, chymotrypsin,

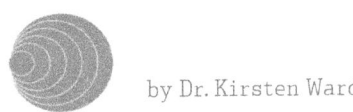

carboxypolypeptidase and elastase). Most of the proteins have been broken down into dipeptides and tripeptides. The final peptide bonds are broken after the molecules have entered the enterocytes (specialized cells) that line the villi of the small intestines. Villi are small projections on the intestinal wall that increase the surface area to aid absorption. Within each of the enterocyte cells there is cytosol (intercellular fluid) which contains multiple other peptidase enzymes that complete the breakdown of all the proteins into the smallest protein particle: the amino acid. It is the amino acid that the body can utilize as needed.

Digestion of fats in the small intestines

There are several digested components that are considered part of the fat group. Phospholipids, cholesterol esters and cholesterol join triglycerides in the fat family. Fats and water do not combine well, so the initial step in fat digestion is to break up the larger units into smaller units through peristalsis in the small intestines (called emulsification). The units then become small enough for liver secretions to break them down further. The liver contributes bile acids in the form of bile salts and lecithin to aid in fat digestion. Both the bile salts and lecithin are amphiphilic (zwitterions) which means they have ends that are different polarities. Water is a polar molecule, whereas fat is a non-polar molecule. Bile salts and lecithin have one end that combines with the fat globule and the other polar end faces outside of the globule to be combined with the polar water molecule. The polar, watery fluid surrounds the fat globule, increasing the tension between its moving particles. This results in the globule further breaking up into smaller components. In the end the fat globules become smaller and smaller. The lipase enzyme is only effective on the surface of the fat molecule. As the surface area of the fat globule increases, the more effective the enzyme can be. The pancreas now contributes some very important enzymes to digest the varieties of fats. Pancreatic lipase works on the triglycerides, cholesterol ester hydrolase works on the cholesterol, and phospholipase A_2 works on phospholipids. At this point most

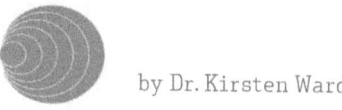

digestion has taken place. It is towards the absorption of these components that we turn our attention.

Absorption occurs through the cell wall of the small intestines. Villi, or small protrusions into the interior of the small intestines, results in a nearly 1000-fold increase in surface area which is equivalent to the entire surface area of a tennis court. (Hall & Guyton, 2011, p. 837)

Digestion of carbohydrates in the small intestines

Most carbohydrates that are utilized within the body are digested into the monosaccharide (single sugar) of glucose (80%) (Hall & Guyton, 2011, p. 839). Glucose and galactose (from milk) are absorbed through the intestinal membrane by a two-part active transport of sodium ions. Active transport means that it takes energy to move both of these types of sugars through the membrane for absorption into the bloodstream. Fructose is absorbed through a facilitated transport method which requires a special membrane proteins to function like a door. Fructose equilibrium is thereby achieved without energy. The rate of equalization within and without the membrane is much slower for fructose than for glucose and galactose, which is what gives fructose the characteristic of a slow sugar absorption or a lack of blood sugar spike.

There are also a number of carbohydrates consumed that do not follow the carbohydrate pathway outlined above. In 2001, The American Association of Cereal Chemists outlined certain carbohydrates as being "resistant to digestion and absorption in the human small intestine." These "included non-starch polysaccharides, such as cellulose, pectin, and gums, as well as resistant oligosaccharides such as fructooligosaccharides and galactooligosaccharides, and other carbohydrates such as resistant starch (RS) and dextrins." In addition, there is "lignin, which is bound to cellulose in the plant cell wall, and some animal origin carbohydrates, such as chitin, hyaluronan, and chondroitin sulfate" (Hamaker & Tuncil, 2014, p. 3839).

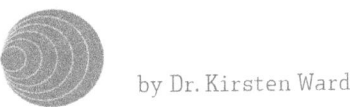

How the body uses Fiber

What does this mean with regard to the foods that we consume? Basically, "cellulose cannot be considered a food for humans." (Hall & Guyton, 2011, p. 833) Instead, we call these fibers.

Recent advances in science have discovered that "[t]he GI tract of healthy animals is colonized by resident populations of microorganisms." Instead of trying to clean out all these organisms we need to learn about what they do. These new discoveries have further found that "[i]n some animals, the gut microbiota contributes directly to nutrition by the fermentative degradation of plant cell-wall polysaccharides." (Karasov & Douglas, 2013, p. 13) This is a mutualistic relationship. The human host benefits from having the nutritional byproduct of the organism and the organism obtains the nutrition through the environment of the host.

The wide variety of foods that support the human have had the added benefit of increasing the number and variety of micro-organisms that live in the GI tract. "…[T]he composition varies widely among individuals, and is influenced by age, diet, and medical condition, including history of orally administered antibiotic treatment." These studies look at fecal matter of the hosts. The analysis has shown how important the diet of the host is to determine the composition and capacity for metabolism based on "whether the host is a carnivore, omnivore or herbivore." (Karasov & Douglas, 2013, p. 14)

"All vertebrates apparently lack the capacity to degrade cellulose and related complex polysaccharides of plant cell walls." If the gastrointestinal tract of humans is working properly and has the correct balance of beneficial microbes then the mutual relationship contributes to the digestion of these otherwise indigestible carbohydrates. Here is what scientists have discovered so far: *Bacteroides* that live in the human colon break up complex polysaccharides into sugars; the sugars are taken in by

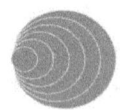
Bifidobacterium and other bacteria and converted into lactate; this lactate is then fermented by other bacteria (*Eubacterium hallii* and *Roseburia hominis*) producing butyrate. Butyrate, which is a waste product of the microbial community, is then used by the intestinal epithelial cells. At least 50% of ingested cellulose and 80% of noncellulosic polysaccharides are converted by microorganisms in the human colon to substances that contribute at least 10% of the human energetic needs. (Karasov & Douglas, 2013, p. 15) Karasov et. al. evaluated vast groups of animals to postulate about how the structure and function of the GI tract work together. Microorganisms in the human body are primarily found in the small and large intestine. This places their colonies after the acidic environment of the stomach. Karasov concluded that this organization offers the opportunity for the microorganism to utilize components that were indigestible to the host human and would "minimize…the competition between animal and resident microorganisms for ingested nutrients that can be processed readily…" (Karasov & Douglas, 2013, p. 16) They confirmed the mutualistic symbiotic relationship between colonizing micro-organisms and the host.

Mutualism between humans and the microbiome

Additional studies have found that the healthy human biome is dominated by four phyla: Firmicutes, Bacteroidetes, Proteobacteria, and Actinobacteria. In order of abundance, Firmicutes and Bacteroidetes are the most abundant, followed by Proteobacteria and Actinobacteria, with a few other varieties, including Verrucomicrobia and Fusobacteria. The gastrointestinal microbiome provides a wide variety of beneficial functions, including: 1) converting indigestible items into nutritional factors that the body can use (vitamins); 2) detoxifying certain ingested items; 3) functioning as an immune system; 4) signaling when epithelial cells need renewing and thereby maintaining the integrity of the gut lining; and 5) providing a competitive environment for other microbial colonies. Linoleic acids, vitamins (e.g. folate, riboflavin), and secondary bile acids, have local and systemic effects

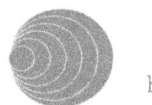

upon the host. These effects include being anti-inflammatory and regulating other metabolic pathways. Most of the primary bile acids are rapidly converted by bacteria into secondary bile acids. Secondary bile acids protect against muscle fat deposition. They also bind to the vitamin D receptor to promote a detoxifying mechanism that protects the host cells against injury and inflammation. At physiological levels, they may even contribute to the regulation of the mucosal barrier functions, cell renewal, and immune function. (Sun & Chang, 2014, p. 133) These are all beneficial to the host and are by-products of the colonizing microorganisms.

The microbial colonization of the intestinal tract starts after birth, and begins with facultative anaerobes (microbes that can survive with and without oxygen) and then by bifidobacteria, clostridia, bacteroides, and other strict anaerobes (microbes that do not need oxygen). Studies have shown that during the first year of life the microflora is very active but has a low diversity. By the time a child has reached the age of 2 or 3 the population has stabilized to resemble that of an adult. (Neu, 2012, p. 94) Current understanding of how hosts recover important nutrients from their microbiota is not complete. Continued investigation is needed to answer the questions: location and quantity of digestive enzymes in the host that contribute to the absorption of essential nutrients that are produced by the microbiome and whether the resultant nutritional products are sufficient to affect the required nutritional needs of the host. (Karasov & Douglas, 2013, p. 41)

How to make fiber more bioavailable to humans

Starch, which is also a type of carbohydrate is semi-crystalline at room temperature but "undergoes crystalline-to-amorphous transformation in water when heated to 60–70°C, which accounts for the various changes of starchy foods when they are cooked." During the cooking process starch chains swell up and can then be more easily digested by the body's hydrolytic enzymes. Cellulose has a similar transformation but requires a "significantly

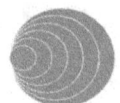

higher temperature." (Deguchi, Tsujii, & Horikoshi, 2006, p. 3293) This indicates that for the body's hydrolytic enzymes to more easily digest cellulose it must be heated and therefore cooked. To get them most out of plant cells that contain cellulose, you must cook them.

Many fruits and vegetables contain another fiber source: pectin. It is "the generic term for a family of galacturonic acid polymers which occur naturally in all plant cell walls, [and] is one of several components of dietary fibre [sic]." (Cummings et al., 1979, p. 477) In a study of normally functioning individuals it was found that "Pectin could not be recovered from the faeces [sic] suggesting that it is totally metabolized in the gut." (Cummings et al., 1979, p. 478) In this article other studies were referenced that demonstrated a high wheat fiber diet "could lead to significant C[alcium] imbalance" (Cummings et al., 1979, p. 484) and that the amount of imbalance could be seen as directly proportional to the uronic acid content of the fiber. Since pectin has a very high uronic acid content Cummings expected to see an imbalance of Calcium. However, this was not the case. The only changes in fecal matter observed were increases in the percentages of "excretion of fatty acids, N[itrogen], bile acids and total solids." The authors concluded that the extra fecal solids combined with the increase in fat and Nitrogen excretions without the effect on the digestion and absorption of these nutrients in the small intestines were the result of "an increase in bacterial mass." (Cummings et al., 1979, p. 484) Fiber "is metabolized by bacteria to short chain fatty acids hydrogen, carbon dioxide and methane." (Cummings et al., 1979, p. 484) In other words, bacteria in the digestive tract were digesting the fiber and releasing their waste products into the human fecal matter. It was the waste products of the bacteria that was equal to the amount of additional pectin in the human diet. Humans have a mutualistic symbiotic relationship with the bacteria in their digestive tract. (Karasov & Douglas, 2013, p. 3)

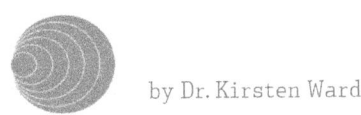

Absorption of Amino Acids in the small intestines

Amino Acid (Protein) absorption is like the glucose absorption, in that energy is required to move the amino acid from one side of the cell membrane to the other. The specific type of channel varies from one amino acid to another. This is the way the body can regulate the precise one of the 20 amino acids it requires. As mentioned before, there are 8-11 essential amino acids. Essential denotes that the body cannot produce them from other components but must obtain them directly from food. The essential amino acids are: histidine, isoleucine, leucine, lysine, methionine, phenylalanine, threonine, tryptophan and valine. The non-essential amino acids are assembled and disassembled by the body as needed. Human muscle tissue is a great source of essential amino acids. Amino acids also require other cofactors, like vitamins and minerals, to aid in their absorption into the body. (Balch, 2010, p. 55) There is a highly delicate balance of required elements to make amino acids bioavailable to the body.

All Amino Acids (with the exception of glycine) are found in the human body in a particular configuration that biologists describe as the L- version. Getting into too much detail is out of the scope of this paper, but a general overview is important for understanding how the body differentiates between the two versions.

The importance of Molecule Configuration

Let us take a closer look at the different configurations of molecules and why this is important to humans. Molecules are L- versus D- and can be understood from the perspective of the difference between a left-handed glove versus a right-handed glove. Each of these gloves is composed of the same parts: a pointer finger, a middle finger, a ring finger, a pinky and a thumb. The difference is in the combination of these parts. You cannot put a left-handed glove onto a right hand or a right-handed glove onto a left hand. The assembly of the parts of the molecule becomes important because of the way the body utilizes it. Biological systems recognize the difference between the right-handed versus the left-handed

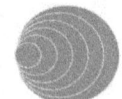

molecules and respond differently to each one. The most famous illustration of this phenomenon is seen in the tragic case of the Thalidomide babies of the late 1950s and very early 1960s (Bernstein & Sullivan, 2015). Thalidomide was a drug that was marketed to pregnant women to help with morning sickness. When the public began using the drug it was not understood how it could affect individuals. It turns out there were two differently handed forms of the compound. One version of the compound produced children who had the characteristic flipper hands and legs while the other version of the compound did not produce any visible deformities. While the body's response to the differently assembled molecules is not always as tragic as that seen by Thalidomide, care must be taken in monitoring how the body does use the different forms. (Nguyen, He, & Pham-Huy, 2006, p. 92)

Amino Acid Configuration

Since a majority of the amino acids are assembled from other amino acids, we will only look closely at the essential ones. Essential amino acids are those that must come directly from food sources. As with the fingers on the glove, all amino acids have similar fingers: ("Threonine Amino Acid," n.d.). The difference of one amino acid from another is in the composition of the part labeled "R" in the image above. Threonine and Isoleucine have two places in which the placement of the components could be assembled in a way that is either left or right handed. This results in four distinct assembly options for these two amino acids. As already mentioned, the human body only utilizes the L- assembly of amino acids for its own uses. Some bacteria are able to utilize the D- assembly of some amino acids. ("Threonine Amino Acid," n.d.) This again points to an opportunity for a mutualistic symbiotic relationship between human hosts and their bacterial colonies.

Let us look at the essential amino acids that the body obtains from ingested proteins one at a time. Histidine, which the body obtains from rice, wheat and rye, is vital for the growth and repair of tissues and the myelin sheaths surrounding nerves. It is instrumental in the

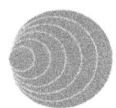

production of both red and white blood cells, helps repair damage from radiation, lowers blood pressure and helps remove heavy metals. Elevated levels of histidine have been shown to lead to stress, anxiety and schizophrenia. (Balch, 2010, p. 61)

Isoleucine, found in almonds, cashews, chicken, chickpeas, eggs, fish, lentils, liver, meat, rye, most seeds and soy, is used by the body to form hemoglobin. Isoleucine along with leucine and valine is a branched-chain amino acid. This is an important observation because they work together synergistically to protect muscle and to act as fuel. Additionally, it stabilizes and regulates blood sugar and energy levels. (Balch, 2010, p. 61)

Leucine together with isoleucine and valine work synergistically in the body to help protect muscle tissue and to act as fuel. Leucine is found in brown rice, beans, meat, nuts, soy, and whole wheat. It also helps in lowering elevated blood sugar levels and in increasing growth hormone production. (Balch, 2010, pp. 61–62)

Lysine, which is found in cheese, eggs, fish, lima beans, milk, potatoes, red meat, soy and yeast, is an essential building block for all proteins. It aids in calcium absorption, and nitrogen balance. In children, it is essential for proper growth as well as bone development. Lysine is also instrumental in producing antibodies, hormones and enzymes. When combined with Vitamin C and bioflavonoids it has been shown to aid the body in fighting off or preventing herpes outbreaks. (Balch, 2010, p. 498)

Methionine, found in beans, eggs, fish, garlic, lentils, meat, onions, soybeans, seeds and yogurt, acts as an antioxidant and is the source of sulfur in the body that inactivates free radicals. It is used to assist in the breakdown of fats and to prevent skin and nail problems. The body uses methionine in every cell to help in the synthesis of nucleic acids, collagen and proteins as well as the other amino acids cysteine and taurine. The body can also use methionine to make choline which is needed by the brain. (Balch, 2010, p. 62)

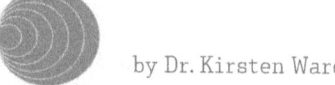

Phenylalanine crosses the blood-brain barrier and therefore can directly affect brain chemistry. The naturally found L- version is found in beef, poultry, pork, fish, milk, yogurt, eggs, cheese, soy, and certain nuts and seeds. The artificial sweetener aspartame is also high in phenylalanine. ("Phenylalanine," n.d.) The D- version, which is a mirror image of the L- version, is made in laboratories and is used to treat pain (especially arthritis) in humans. The L- form is used by the body as a building block for proteins. It can also be converted into another amino acid, tyrosine, which the body uses in the brain to make the neurotransmitters dopamine and norepinephrine. These two neurotransmitters are what the body uses to promote alertness and thereby influence memory and learning. Interestingly, they also support appetite suppression. (Balch, 2010, pp. 62–63)

Threonine is found in watercress, spirulina, wild game, turkey, fish, eggs, and soy ("Foods highest in Threonine," n.d.). It is responsible for maintaining a proper balance of protein in the body. In this capacity, it also contributes to the formation of collagen, elastin, and tooth enamel and aids the liver in fat metabolism with the help of the other amino acids: aspartic acid and methionine. The body stores threonine in the heart, central nervous system and skeletal muscle. When the body is in need of mounting an immune response, threonine is used to help produce antibodies. Additionally, threonine can be used by the body to make the other amino acids: glycine and serine. (Balch, 2010, p. 63)

Tryptophan is found in brown rice, cottage cheese, meat, peanuts and soy. This amino acid is extremely important for the neurotransmitter serotonin. It is serotonin that the brain uses to help promote nerve impulses from one cell to another. Tryptophan has been seen to help with hyperactivity in children as well as stress management in adults. Additionally, it is given credit for heart health, weight control and the release of growth hormone. Tryptophan is required for B_3 (niacin) production. The co-factors

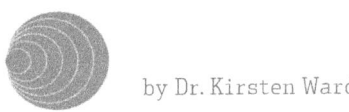

that the body needs to utilize tryptophan are vitamins B$_6$ (pyridoxine), and C, folate and magnesium. (Balch, 2010, p. 64)

The last of the essential amino acids is valine. It is found in dairy products, grains, meat, mushrooms, peanuts and soy. Valine is the last of the trio of branched amino acids: isoleucine and leucine. These three must always be balanced for optimal health. The body stores valine in the muscle tissues and can draw from it when there is an increased need for energy. Valine is used by the body for stimulant effects, metabolism of muscle, tissue repair and maintenance of nitrogen balance. (Balch, 2010, p. 64)

Essential Fatty Acids

The absorption of fats is very straightforward. The cell membranes are constructed of fatty acid heads with phospholipid tails which blend with the zwitterion glycerol and fatty acids that have been digested in the duodenum and upper jejunum. Short and medium chain fatty acids can be absorbed directly into the blood stream without going through more digestion.

The two essential fatty acids (EFAs) for human beings are Linoleic Acid and Alpha-Linolenic Acid. Both must be obtained from the food eaten since the body is not able to manufacture them. Alpha-Linoleic Acid is found in flax, hemp, canola, soy, walnut and dark leafy greens and Linoleic Acid is found in safflower, sunflower, hemp soy, walnut, pumpkin, sesame, and flax oil. (Erasmus, 1993, pp. 21–22) EFAs have the special qualities of attracting oxygen, absorbing sunlight and carrying a slightly negative charge (unusual for nonpolar fats). (Erasmus, 1993, p. 45) These qualities enable EFAs to be used by the body for energy production, oxygen transfer, hemoglobin production, component of cell membranes, fatigue recovery, prostaglandin precursor (hormone-like substance in the body), growth, and cell division just to name a few. (Erasmus, 1993, pp. 46–51)

Vitamins and Minerals

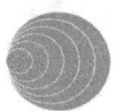

Vitamins and minerals are micronutrients that help the body regulate metabolism and assist the biochemical processes that release energy from digested food. They are "essential to life". (Balch, 2010, p. 18) Since both vitamins and minerals have been studied almost exclusively as individual elements and not as parts of actually consumed foods, we will only take a cursory look at them. This area of nutrition is constantly evolving, but the essential understanding is: the body has a constant need for quality and variety of foods to supply all micronutrients that support life.

Vitamins

Vitamins have been described as coming in two major classes: Water Soluble and Oil Soluble varieties. Water soluble ones go through the entire body in four to twenty-four hours and are therefore required every day. These are Vitamin C, and the B Complex.

Vitamin C, also known as Ascorbic Acid, is found in berries, citrus fruits and green vegetables. It is an antioxidant that is involved in at least three hundred metabolic functions in the body. Vitamin E and beta-carotene are necessary to optimally utilize the benefits of Vitamin C. Depletion of vitamin C in the body can occur when an individual indulges in alcohol consumption, pain killers, antidepressants, blood thinners, oral contraceptives, steroids and smoking. (Balch, 2010, p. 26)

The B complex vitamins are also water soluble and are comprised of several members. Together they help the nerves, skin, eyes, hair, liver and mouth as well as muscle tone in the gastrointestinal tract and proper brain function. The entire group is comprised of B_1 (Thiamine), B_2 (Riboflavin), B_3 (Niacin), B_5 (Pantothenic Acid), B_6 (Pyridoxine), B_{12} (Methylcobalamin), Biotin, Choline, Folate, Inositol and Para-Aminobenzoic Acid (PABA). These are so crucial to health and wellbeing that many processed foods are supplemented with them. "Enriched" wheat products have been supplemented with B-complex vitamins. (Balch, 2010, pp. 20–26)

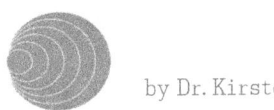

Oil soluble vitamins can be stored in the body's fatty tissue and in the liver. As such they are not needed as frequently as the water-soluble vitamins. Vitamins A, D, E, and K belong to this group. All the oil soluble vitamins require fat to aid in the digestion and absorption. (Neu, 2012, p. 137) Additionally, they all go through the liver and therefore require an optimally functioning liver.

Vitamin A "refers to a number of compounds that include both the naturally occurring and synthetically derived retinoids." (Neu, 2012, p. 137) Your vision, growth, healing, reproduction, cell differentiation, immunocompetency, healthy skin and barrier functions are a result of good Vitamin A levels. How does the body use Vitamin A for all these various functions? "The action is similar to that of steroid hormones in that a specific retinoic acid receptor protein complex becomes bound to nuclear DNA, resulting in regulation of specific genes." In this way Vitamin A has been credited with regulating more than 500 genes. (Neu, 2012, p. 137) In combination the vitamin A compounds have been shown to be more beneficial than single Vitamin A carotenoids taken individually. (Balch, 2010, p. 19) Add to the picture that not all of the carotenoids have been discovered, and it becomes clear that obtaining Vitamin A should ideally come from actual food sources. "Animal sources of vitamin A are up to six times as strong as vegetable sources…"(Balch, 2010, p. 20) Vitamin A is carried in the plasma and synthesized in the liver. Some Vitamin A compounds are converted to useful components in the small intestines with the help of secretions from the liver. Bile salts combined with the Vitamin A compounds and are then absorb into the small intestines and are stored in the liver (90% of body stores). (Neu, 2012, p. 137)

Vitamin D has properties that are characteristic of both a vitamin and a hormone and is required for the absorption and utilization of calcium and phosphorus. There are several sources of this vitamin: a food source, a sunlight source and a synthetic source. The food source of Vitamin D is not fully active and, as with the other oil soluble vitamins, requires conversion by the liver with contributions

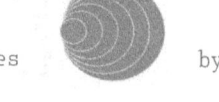 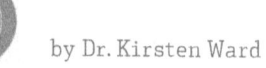

of the kidneys. (Balch, 2010, p. 27) Research on Vitamin D is currently ongoing. Suffice it to say that obtaining Vitamin D from natural sources is the best alternative.

As with the other oil soluble vitamins, Vitamin E is a family of compounds. It is found in avocados, cold-pressed vegetable oils, dark leafy vegetables, legumes, nuts, seeds and whole grains, among others. Vitamin E is crucial for the utilization of all the other oil soluble compounds because it helps prevent them from destruction by oxygen. The liver carefully selects for the absorption of Vitamin E. Absorption is also influenced by zinc and Vitamin C levels. (Balch, 2010, pp. 28–29)

Vitamin K comes in three recognized forms: K_1 from food sources, K_2 is made in the small intestines by the colonizing bacteria and from some food sources (butter, cow liver, chicken, eggs fermented soy and cheese), K_3 is a humanly synthesized compound. Most of the body's supply of Vitamin K comes from the bacteria that colonize the small intestines. The liver is responsible for extracting the Vitamin K from the bacterial by-products. Vitamin K is responsible for blood clotting factors and bone tissue repair and maintenance. (Balch, 2010, p. 30) Vitamin K is absorbed from the intestine into the lymphatic system, requiring the presence of both bile salts and pancreatic secretions. (Neu, 2012, p. 142) As we have previously mentioned, necessary compounds in the body work together. As such, it is not surprising that Vitamin K requires the aid of calcium for optimal functioning. (Balch, 2010, p. 30)

Bioflavonoids and Coenzyme Q_{10} can be added to the Vitamin section (See (Balch, 2010, pp. 30–31)), but are not considered true vitamins. Bioflavonoids work synergistically with Vitamin C and are not produced by the body. Together they support strong capillary strength. Coenzyme Q_{10} is one of a group of ten antioxidants designated as coenzyme Q but only the Q_{10} is found in human tissue. It has a strong anti-aging effect and aids in circulation and immunity.

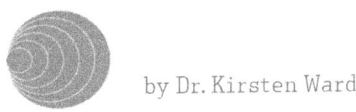

Minerals

Minerals are also extremely important for life. The human body works best in the chemical balances of the interactions of vitamins, minerals, water and the carbs, fats, proteins. Minerals like calcium, sulfur, sodium, potassium and phosphorus are needed in larger quantities. Some trace minerals include magnesium, silicon, fluorine, strontium, chromium, copper, iodine, iron, manganese, molybdenum, selenium, nickel, cobalt, vanadium, boron, germanium, and zinc. As with oil soluble vitamins, minerals can be stored in the body. Unlike the liver storage of oil soluble vitamins, however, minerals are stored in bone and muscle. (Balch, 2010, p. 32)

We will take a brief look at some of these minerals to get an idea of how the body uses them. Calcium is widely known to be important for strong bones, teeth and healthy gums. It also provides energy, maintains regular heartbeat, and supports nerve impulses. There are many foods that contain calcium, but the challenge for the human body to use calcium comes in two forms: the complex relationship between calcium absorption with the many required cofactors (especially magnesium and phosphorus) and the tremendous amount of calcium the body requires. (Balch, 2010, p. 33)

Sulfur is an acid forming mineral and is found in the essential amino acid, Methionine. (Balch, 2010, p. 42)

Sodium combined with potassium is responsible for the sodium/potassium pump on the membranes of each and every cell in the body. This pump controls the correct acid/alkaline environment inside and outside of the cells. Together sodium and potassium maintain the proper blood pH and water balance in the body. (Balch, 2010, p. 41)

Silicon levels decrease with age and have been shown to influence the negative effects of aluminum on the body. Protection from Alzheimer's disease has been seen from sustained higher levels of

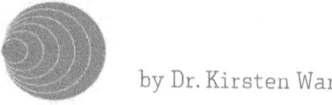

silicon in older individuals. Other minerals that need to be in correct balance for silicon to work optimally are boron, calcium, magnesium, manganese and potassium. (Balch, 2010, p. 41)

Copper, zinc and vitamin C must exist in balance to obtain the optimal utilization of all three. Elevated copper levels result in reduced levels of vitamin C and zinc while elevated zinc and vitamin C levels reduce the copper levels. Copper aids in bone formation, hemoglobin and red blood cells. (Balch, 2010, p. 36) Zinc balances the absorption of vitamins A and E. It is also important for the reproductive organs. Eating foods containing phytates (found in grains and legumes) has been shown to bind with zinc and prevent the body from being able to utilize it. (Balch, 2010, p. 43)

Iodine is an important mineral for the metabolism of excess fat and for physical and mental development. The body uses iodine in the thyroid to help with thyroid hormone secretions. Foods that are grown near the coasts contain more iodine than those grown inland. (Balch, 2010, p. 37)

Iron is an absolutely critical nutrient for many biological processes. The most important process is for the formation of red blood cells and hemoglobin production (other processes iron is critical for are: DNA replication, gene expression, cell respiration, and the transport and delivery of oxygen). It is an important component of many enzymes essential for brain development and for cardiac and skeletal muscle function (myoglobin). (Neu, 2012, p. 145) The body obtains iron from both organic and inorganic forms. The organic form is highly absorbable by the human body (bioavailable) and is found in the liver and muscle of red meat. The inorganic form is much less bioavailable and can be influenced by dietary factors including phytates, phosphates, tannates, oxalates, and carbonates. (Neu, 2012, p. 145) When the human body does not have sufficient iron, it is able to prioritize the available iron both between and within organs. (Neu, 2012, p. 148) To make the situation even more complicated, uptake of iron is influenced by hydrochloric acid levels in the

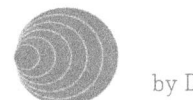

stomach as well as body levels of copper, manganese, molybdenum, vitamin A, the B-complexes, vitamin C, zinc, vitamin E and calcium levels.

Enzymes

Enzymes have been called the "sparks of life" (Dr. Edward Howell) and function by lowering the energy of activation required for a chemical process to take place. Each enzyme is required for a specific chemical reaction and is therefore, irreplaceable. Without enzymes, the chemical reactions would take place too slowly for life to exist. At this point in science they have distinguished two types of enzymes important to humans: digestive and metabolic. "[T]he functions of enzymes are so many and so diverse that it would be impossible to name them all." (Balch, 2010, p. 72)

There are basically three kinds of digestive enzymes: amylase, protease and lipase. All three of these should be familiar by now, since they were previously described during the digestion process.

Metabolic enzymes are responsible for activities of all the body's organs, tissues and cells. While the body is able to manufacture enzymes as needed, it should obtain them from foods also. Enzymes are sensitive to heat and therefore should come from raw foods.

The Large Intestine and Colon

As a final stop in our journey through the digestive tract of human beings, we must take a quick look at the large intestine and colon. This area of the tract is responsible for recycling water and for holding waste until elimination is possible. The large intestine is responsible for absorbing 6 to 7 liters of water and mixing the remainder with fecal matter. (Hall & Guyton, 2011, p. 840) "Without adequate water, we would poison ourselves with our own metabolic wastes." (Balch, 2010, p. 47)

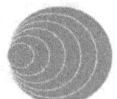

Struggles with a dysfunctioning Digestive Tract

As previously mentioned, the majority of individuals who come in for Thermograms suffer from digestive disorders. These can show up as any combination of: physiological compensation (acid and alkaline imbalance), food intolerance, sensitivity, dysbiosis (mycosis or bacterial infection) and putrification. All living things consume for the purposes of maintaining the body and for energy. Human beings have invented an entire market of "non-food" items that we ingest. These non-food items include highly processed substances that are marketed as food items. They vary in their ability to provide building blocks for the body to use in maintenance and to provide energy for function. "The fuel we give our bodies' engines comes directly from the things we consume. The foods we eat contain nutrients. These nutrients come in the form of vitamins, minerals, enzymes, water, amino acids, carbohydrates and lipids." (Balch, 2010, p. 3)

pH imbalance in the Digestive Tract

When there is an acid and alkaline imbalance in the gastrointestinal tract, the result is an inability of the body to obtain the nutrients from the consumed foods. Throughout the entire tract, the body carefully controls the pH levels to produce the desired outcomes for digestion and absorption. Enzyme activity is extremely specific and when imbalance exists a whole cascade of further imbalances occur in the body. This is easily explained by the previous discussion of the interrelated chemical processes.

For a body exhibiting a need for support due to physiologically compensated signature patterns, the absorption and utilization of Amino Acids becomes extremely important. An imbalance in acid and alkalinity changes the charge of the solvents within the digestive tract. Each area of the digestive track has a different pH depending upon what is being digested and absorbed. For example, the ideal human saliva has a pH of 6.4 and readily breaks down carbohydrates, while the stomach acid ideally has a pH of 1.5 to 3.0

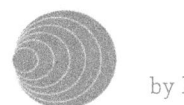

(Haldiman, MS, & RN, 2013) which is designed to begin the breakdown of proteins into the amino acid building blocks. The extreme environment of the stomach underscores the challenge of breaking down these proteins and the amount of energy the human body exerts to achieve this task. Every amino acid is composed of one amino group, one carboxyl group, and the R group. "Amino acids have the property of being charged as positive (α amino group) one negative (α carboxyl group) depending on the pH of the solution" (Litwack, 2008, p. 46). Of the 20 essential amino acids, 13 have two ionizable groups but the remaining 7 amino acids have three. (Litwack, 2008, p. 48) What does this mean for the individual who has a physiologically compensated signature pattern? When this condition exists, the amino acids that have the amino group, the carboxyl group or the R group with pronated or depronated ends will not be available to the body as they are needed. Specifically the enzyme pepsin in the stomach, is most active at a pH of 2.0 to 3.0 and is rendered inactive at a pH above 5.0. This means that when the pH is off there is a possibility that a person might not be able to digest proteins at all. (Hall & Guyton, 2011, pp. 840)

When the body is in need of amino acids, it will redirect those amino acids from muscle tissue, where the body stores them, to support the liver and heart during times of poor intake. "Insufficient intake of vitamins and minerals, especially vitamin C, can interfere with the absorption of amino acids in the lower part of the small intestines. Vitamin B_6 is needed also…." (Balch, 2010, p. 55) Low levels of isoleucine have been found to cause symptoms similar to hypoglycemia and several mental and physical disorders. (Balch, 2010, p. 61) Recall that this amino acid is found in four different assemblages. The human body only uses one of the four. Insufficient levels of lysine are seen to result in anemia, bloodshot eyes, enzyme disorders, hair loss, inability to concentrate, irritability, lack of energy, poor appetite, reproductive disorders, retarded growth and weight loss. There is no mention of elevated methionine levels in individuals, rather, "it is wise to supplement the diet with choline or lecithin to ensure that the supply of methionine is not depleted."

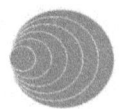

(Balch, 2010, p. 62) When the body is deficient in Threonine, the person may exhibit symptoms like: irritability, lack of energy, poor appetite, or inability to concentrate. Physical symptoms may include bloodshot eyes, loss of hair, retarded growth, and weight loss. (Hawwa, 2015) Low levels of tryptophan result in Niacin deficiencies and have been shown to range from the mild symptoms: indigestion, fatigue, canker sores, vomiting and depression; to more severe symptoms of pellagra. Pellagra is a disease that is characterized by thick, scaly pigmented rash on skin that is exposed to sunlight, swollen mouth and bright red tongue, vomiting and diarrhea, headache, apathy, fatigue, depression, disorientation memory loss. If not treated, it will lead to a premature death. ("Niacin Deficiency," n.d.) Low histidine levels require not only increased histidine, but also vitamins B_3 (Niacin) and B_6 (Pyridoxine) to help transform histidine into histamine. It is the histamine that is responsible for improved sexual functioning and pleasure as well as stimulating the secretion of gastric juices. (Balch, 2010, p. 61)

On the vitamin front low levels resulting from either lack of consumption or the body's inability to extract them from foods can result in a variety of symptoms. The deficiency of vitamin C results in poor wound healing, soft and spongy bleeding gums, edema, extreme weakness, and "pinpoint" hemorrhages under the skin and is called Scurvy. (Balch, 2010, p. 26) In an article presented in the American Journal of Medical Sciences, Singh, et. al. described "Evidence [that] suggests....recognizing scurvy...is...an underdiagnosed ailment in the developed world." (Singh, Richards, Lykins, Pfister, & McClain, 2015, p. 373) Other "[s]tudies have shown that at least 40 percent of people have less-than-optimal levels of the vitamin [D] in their blood." This statistic is even higher in the Hispanic and Black sub-populations. (Balch, 2010, p. 27) It has been found that only 8 percent of men and 2.4 percent of women in the United States consume the government recommended amounts of vitamin E. Since we know that the government gives minimum requirements, it is safe to say that there is a vitamin E

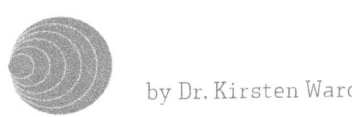

deficiency across the board in the United States. Ingested vitamin E is not easily absorbed by the body. Deficiency of vitamin E results in damage to red blood cells, infertility (in both men and women), menstrual problems, neuromuscular impairment, shortened life span of red blood cells, miscarriages and uterine degeneration, impaired balance and coordination. (Balch, 2010, pp. 28–29) Deficiencies in Vitamin K are associated with insulin and glucose regulation problems, as well as low bone density in women. (Balch, 2010, p. 30)

Gastrointestinal Dysbiosis

Dysbiosis, broadly defined, is "any change to the composition of resident commensal communities relative to the community found in healthy individuals." (Petersen & Round, 2014, p. 1028) It can increase the risk of disease when the delicate balance between the bacterial community, host and microbiota are disrupted. Petersen & Round continue to describe how commonly used antibiotics have long lasting effects on the microbiota of the human GI tract. "These include (i) loss of beneficial microbial organisms, (ii) expansion of…potentially harmful microorganisms and (iii) loss of overall microbial diversity." (Petersen & Round, 2014, p. 1029) Each of these effects can exist alone or in combination. Sun & Chang describe how dysbiosis can become a chronic problem: 1) the dysbiosis activates the host immune and inflammation response; 2) a disruption in the previous homeostasis of the intestines is achieved; 3) the organisms that colonized in a harsher environment increase in number thereby contributing to continued inflammatory response; 4) the continued inflammatory response prevents the beneficial organisms from recolonizing. Taken together these create a chronically diseased state. (Sun & Chang, 2014, p. 133) Inflammation is the body's response to invaders and should not be seen as something to be totally eradicated. It is an immune reaction, that (like a fever) is a double-edged sword. "[H]ost health depends on a balance between too much proinflammatory activation (leading to tissue injury and clinical sequelae) and not enough (leaving

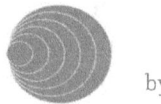

mucosa undefended or poised to self-destruct)" (Neu, 2012, p. 79-80)

Fungus and Virus in the Digestive Tract

In addition to the bacterial microbiome there exists fungal and viral members found in the human GI tract. Petersen & Round described how these three groups can wreak havoc on a host organism: "antibiotic treatment can allow for outgrowth of fungal species in the gut that can influence extra-intestinal disease within the host. Viral members of our microbiota are only just beginning to be identified." (Petersen & Round, 2014, p. 1029) What happens to this community of imbalance when it continues unchecked is described by Neu: "If this self-perpetuating avalanche cannot be stopped, the inflammatory reaction in the gut will drive the development of SIRS, sepsis, and septic shock with associated multiorgan failure (MOF) and death." (Neu, 2012, p. 298) How to change and influence the human microbiome for healing and beneficial outcomes is currently an important area of research. We will only take a brief look at it when we discuss supplementation.

When there is either a malabsorption or a digestion issue, enzymes can be difficult to obtain from raw foods. (Balch, 2010, p. 73) Providing the body with the building blocks to manufacture the enzymes it requires is a good way to achieve the goal of healing without taxing the digestive tract further. Additionally, some foods when eaten raw block the uptake of iodine into the thyroid and should be avoided. (These include Brussel sprouts, cabbage, cauliflower, kale, peaches, pears, spinach and turnips.) (Balch, 2010, p. 37) Cooking foods makes their components more bioavailable.

How the Body Tries to Accommodate Deficiencies

The "triage theory," as proposed by Bruce Ames, describes what adjustments the body makes to accommodate a diet in which there is dysfunction in digestion and therefore an inability to obtain the nutrients from digested food. "[A]s a consequence of a higher need

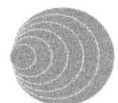

or low intake, micronutrients are delivered from tissues to other organs depending on their need, and priority is given to survival." (Biesalski & Tinz, 2017, p. 77) So the body will move micronutrients around in order to address a hierarchy of need. When the core heart and brain function is in need, micronutrients are diverted from the organs and organ systems lower on the hierarchy. The result is that symptoms of nutrient deficiency become apparent. Additional evidence of a body attempting to conserve necessary nutrients is seen in the diversion of the crucial iron stores within the body. When there is an iron deficiency, the iron that is stored in the liver is depleted first, followed by skeletal muscle and the intestine. Once these areas have been depleted of iron, cardiac iron is compromised, followed by brain iron and finally red cell iron. From this list, you can clearly see that once a blood test returns a deficiency in blood levels of iron, the liver, skeletal muscles, intestine and cardiac iron has already been depleted. (Neu, 2012, p. 148)

Essential Fatty Acid deficiencies can also occur. The symptoms of these deficiencies include: eczema-like skin eruptions, loss of hair, liver degeneration, behavior disturbances, kidney degeneration, excessive water loss through the skin accompanied by thirst, drying up of glands, susceptibility to infections, failure of wound healing, sterility in males, miscarriage in females, arthritis-like conditions, heart and circulatory problems, growth retardation, weakness, impairment of vision and learning ability, lack of motor coordination, tingling sensations in arms and legs, behavior changes, high triglycerides, high blood pressure, sticky platelets, tissue inflammation, edema, dry skin, mental deterioration, low metabolic rate, and some kinds of immune dysfunction. (Erasmus, 1993, pp. 44–45) The long-term consequences of micronutrient deficits combined with an inability to correct the problem when it presents itself cause increased health costs and decreased wellness among people. We need to recognize that in the developed world we are not immune to micronutrient deficiencies.

The Supplement Industry

Modern medicine has devised a whole industry of supplementation. The Dietary Supplement Health and Education Act of 1994 defines a Dietary Supplement as:

> A product (other than tobacco) that is intended to supplement the diet and that bears or contains one or more of the following dietary ingredients:
>
> (A) a vitamin,
>
> (B) a mineral,
>
> (C) a herb or other botanical,
>
> (D) an amino acid,
>
> (E) a dietary substance for use by humans to supplement the diet by increasing the total dietary intake,
>
> (F) a concentrate, metabolite, constituent, extract, or combination of any of these ingredients. (Gardiner et al., 2008, p. 963)

This definition of dietary supplement does not differentiate between the minimally processed whole food micronutrients or pharmaceutically processed active ingredients described as individual micronutrients.

For the purposes of this paper we will differentiate between two major classes of supplements. There are supplements that are derived of whole foods and have minimal processing, or there are supplements that are derived from active ingredients that have either been chemically manufactured in a lab or removed from a whole food. If supplements are produced from minimally processed foods,

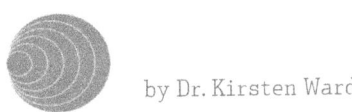

then those supplements contain other components of those food sources that might be yet undiscovered. These undiscovered components have unknown characteristics, but that does not prevent them from being important contributors to human health. Even though the argument has been made that science has "proven" individual "active" ingredients are important. Discoveries of "new" active ingredients are made regularly. As a society, we never know where the discovery is going to come from. Suffice it to say that most discoveries come from an analysis of naturally occurring substances. If the active ingredient is manufactured in a laboratory, then the "synthetic supplements contain the isolated vitamins only" (Balch, 2010, p. 18). In the history of the existence of life on the planet, the existence of vitamins, minerals or enzymes in isolation is a very recent development.

In 2010, the US Department of Agriculture/Department of Health and Human Services outlined some Dietary Guidelines for Americans. In this paper they acknowledge that "supplements containing combinations of certain nutrients may be beneficial in reducing the risks of some chronic diseases when used by special populations." The paper goes on to state that excessive use of certain supplements has the potential to be harmful. More recently, it is estimated that consuming "within the range of two standard deviations above the EAR [estimated average requirement] will not only prevent a deficiency but also cover differences within the individual need." Additionally the published guidelines is seen as a minimum. Anything consumed below that threshold would be seen as "inadequate and places the individual at risk to develop a real deficiency" (Biesalski & Tinz, 2017, p. 77)

Some of these supplements have been associated with potentially negative consequences when taken to excess. "This might in particular be the case for single supplements in concentrations exceeding the normal recommended dietary allowance (RDA), as recently documented, or those with an imbalanced composition." (Biesalski & Tinz, 2017, p. 76)

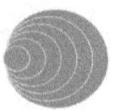

For minerals: Toxic levels can be reached if extremely large quantities are consumed. Additional consideration must be made to the fact that minerals compete with one another for absorption. "[M]inerals should always be taken in balanced amounts." (Balch, 2010, p. 32) For amino acid supplementation: Too much leucine could result in symptoms of hypoglycemia, niacin deficiency and increased ammonia (Balch, 2010, pp. 61–62) Phenylalanine supplementation has been used to influence arthritis pain, depression, menstrual cramps, migraines, obesity, Parkinson's disease and schizophrenia. (Balch, 2010, pp. 62–63) An overabundance of Valine can result in a crawling sensation on the skin and possibly hallucinations. (Balch, 2010, p. 64)

Regardless of where the supplements are derived, in the case of a less than optimally functioning digestive tract, absorption of these micronutrients becomes problematic. Increasing the amount of supplementation enables the body to digest more of the specific micronutrient. The digestion, however, does not ensure bioavailability. This excessive digestion results in a taxing of the liver without the benefit of absorption and ultimate utilization. Additionally, elevated levels can produce unwanted dysfunction as already mentioned. (Balch, 2010, p. 32). "A major problem in understanding the effect of micronutrients is that the body's physiological need is not fully understood across all organs and systems." (Biesalski & Tinz, 2017, p. 77)

It has been suggested that supplementation can be beneficial for the short term "We need to understand that poor diet quality and poor diet diversity are some of the major reasons for micronutrient inadequacies" (Biesalski & Tinz, 2017, p. 78) However, they caution that "A diet with poor quality and an unhealthy lifestyle can never be compensated by any supplement." (Biesalski & Tinz, 2017, p. 80) So then the question becomes: Who should supplement and why? "Generally spoken micronutrients can compensate inadequate supply or transient micronutrient gaps….[I]n cases of sudden disease or periods of inadequate dietary diversity a supplement

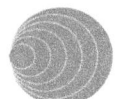
reduces the risk for micronutrient gaps" (Biesalski & Tinz, 2017, p. 80) Biesalski's group concluded that micronutrient gaps happen over time and that the impact on the long term health of the individual would depend on the severity and length of the gap. Their bottom line is: "MVM [Multivitamin and Mineral] supplement consumption has been shown to reduce dietary intake gaps and....can help to counteract potential health issues caused by inadequacy" (Biesalski & Tinz, 2017, p. 81) Basically take supplements when needed, for a short time as a potential preventative measure. The question then becomes: What kind of supplement? I would contend that it should be a whole food supplement, not a single active ingredient one. Let us look at why this would be a beneficial recommendation.

Natural Supplements

Botany, the study of plants, is extremely involved. When studying plants and herbs, researchers have two major problems: 1) once a promising plant is found, it is sometimes over-studied and 2) plants are incredibly complicated from a chemical standpoint. "One of the biggest mistakes researchers make is always trying to fit herbal medicines into a drug model." Dr. Tiera Low Dog says. Modern medical doctors are "so used to looking for one agent — one compound that will do one specific thing in the body, [but] Plants don't typically work that way because they have hundreds of compounds that are very complex, and they're kind of messy to work with...." ("AThymeToHeal.pdf," n.d., p. 148) Regardless of the complexity of plants, this is the method of healing that humans have been using for centuries. Just because it is difficult to quantify in scientific study terms, does not mean the treatments are not valid. The physicians need "to trade the pill-for-an-ill model for one involving maintaining health through proper diet and using natural supplements to treat chronic conditions."("AThymeToHeal.pdf," n.d., p. 148)

Western societies are more cynical when it comes to whether herbal/plant based treatments are effective. "The first thing people

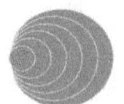

usually ask about…medicinal plants is: Do they work?" (Moerman, 2009, p. 12) Moerman who published an ethnobotanical study of Native American medicinal plants looked into this matter. He decided that the answer to this question had a short answer and a long answer. The short answer was, "yes, they work." But it was the long answer that illustrated an interesting phenomenon in modern society. Here is what he discovered:

> What does it mean to say that a medicine "works"? Essentially it means that the medicine has the effect that we want it to have, that it meets our expectations. This means that a drug that meets one person's expectations may not meet another's, and people may therefore disagree over whether the drug works. Such disagreements usually hinge on different conceptions of health or healing. This is to say that definitions of health and well-being are often cultural matters; they are rarely simple matters of fact. (Moerman, 2009, p. 12)

In other words, "civilized cultures" have a different expectation of their efficacy of treatments. Looking at a longer timeframe than that of the past hundred years of large pharmacological advances in the "civilized world," we can find a rich and varied tradition of humans using herbal and botanical remedies to cure a variety of ailments with great success.

Over the centuries, human traditions have developed the knowledge and use of medicinal plants. Some of the oldest traditions in natural healing are Ayurveda and Traditional Chinese Medicine (TCM). Each of these traditions has histories that stretch over several millennia. "The Chinese Pharmacopoeia (2015, edition) records a total of 644 species of medicinal plants. The recently published Zhong Hua Ben Cao records 8980 Chinese medicinal materials including 7815 herbal substances." (Jaiswal et al., 2016, p. 246) "Ayurveda is the most ancient [of Indian traditional medicine], and most widely accepted and practiced." (Mukherjee, 2001a, 2001b). "Out of the total 17,000–18000 flowering plants species

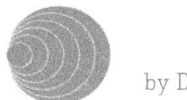

grown in the country, about 7000 species find their usage documented in the folklore medicine of all the five traditional systems of medicines (TSM) of India." (Jaiswal et al., 2016, p. 246) With such impressive traditions it seems short sighted to negate their effectiveness because they do not fit into the "civilized societies'" scientific boxes.

Conclusion

During the discussion on digestion and absorption we looked at the benefits and challenges to each of the major food components: carbohydrates, fats, proteins. In the discussion of carbohydrates, we further went into detail about the variety of indigestible fiber components and their uses for the gastrointestinal tract microbiomes. Recall we discovered cooking provides the opportunity to make some of these fibers more bioavailable for the individual. Similarly, "[E]ncapsulated herbs can be more difficult to digest and assimilate than simple teas and extracts." (Fritchey, 2004, p. 37)

"Nature's healing plants are there and waiting, all around us. They always have been." (Fritchey, 2004, p. 39) Additionally, "[i]n western society, we do think of medicines and food differently." (Pedersen, 1994, p. 1) This picture becomes challenging for certain food items that have clear and strong medicinal qualities. One such food is garlic. "You can buy garlic in the produce section of the market right next to onions and celery. Studies have shown that garlic lowers blood cholesterol levels, reduces blood pressure and kills bacteria. These are medicinal qualities." (Pedersen, 1994, p. 1) So where do we put garlic: Is it a food or a medicine. While this is a very good question, I believe the question is not as important as the question of how we look at food and what we do with it for healing purposes.

Anything put into the body for the purpose of achieving a particular outcome can be considered medicinal. If the goal is to control the symptoms of a body attempting to regain balance, then the medicinal uses of "natural" or man-made pharmaceuticals is still

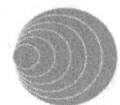

viewed in the realm of allopathic medicine and does not focus on the root causes of the source of the symptom. "[H]erbs can control symptoms [and]…are often chosen…because they are "natural," and therefore assumed "safer"…. The often-forgotten Natural Health axiom that "suppressing symptoms does not heal," is just as true with herbs as it is with allopathic medicine." (Fritchey, 2004, p. 63) Countries that are consumed with the idea of controlling the symptoms need to refocus their efforts on restoring health by providing the body with what it needs and this takes a paradigm shift. "In order to employ herbs to their true advantage – the ability to support the body's effort to heal itself – we must learn to think of the body's actions – its symptoms - and the herb's actions, in synchronistic or synergistic terms." (Fritchey, 2004, p. 63)

"By working with the Natural processes instead of fighting them, we can empower and expedite the resolution of dis-ease, and the restoration of health." (Fritchey, 2004, p. 63) Because herbs are plants and are therefore considered in the realm of food science, we will take a quick look at the chemical complexity of food. So far, we have looked at the basic food elements of fats, proteins, carbohydrates, vitamins, minerals and enzymes because that is how science has categorized the digestive process. Natural foods are complex combinations of a multitude of chemical substances. A simple potato "contains over a hundred and fifty known chemical substances and many unknown chemical substances as well." (Pedersen, 1994, p. 3) Pedersen goes on to explain that "[a]ll natural foods contain substances which affect the structure of function of the body. Most contain about…0.1%. Thus all natural foods have some medicinal action….In fact, the only foods which do not contain these substances are refined foods like white flour and white sugar." (Pedersen, 1994, p. 3) For us this means that eating a wide variety of food items that are minimally refined provides the most usable and beneficial nutrients for our body to make what it needs to repair and run our daily functions. One of the easiest ways to add a variety of nutrients to your diet is to add herbs to your cooking.

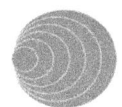

With the ubiquity of Alkaline water in the marketplace, I feel it necessary to provide some observations. The body is constantly monitoring and balancing fluids, functions and actions with the building blocks that the individual provides for it. The choices we make on what we put into our bodies directly provides those available building blocks for the body to use. "The concept of cultivating a more alkaline diet is dismissed in some circles because it's well-known that the human body aggressively regulates the pH of its fluids, regardless of what we put into our mouths. However, our food choices do have an impact on digestion, nutrient absorption, and elimination." (Rubin, 2015, p. 54) We really are what we eat. Our bodies cannot obtain building blocks from things that we do not make available to it.

"Your body is your very best friend. It never leaves you, and even when you think it betrays you, it generally does not....It's absolutely doing everything to adapt and try to survive, given how you care for it. And if you think of your body as your best friend, my guess is that you'll treat it much differently." ("AThymeToHeal.pdf," n.d., p. 150)

On the practitioner side, we need to be the change we want to see. We have a strong position to affect the change in how doctors/practitioners relate to their patients/clients. "[B]efore I look at your labs and test results, I need to hear your story....[g]ood doctors are like good detectives. If you tell us your story, we can often get a good picture of what's going on." ("AThymeToHeal.pdf," n.d., p. 149)

Western and allopathic medicine is first rate in the "acute care model." It does not fare so well with chronic problems that can be "caused or worsened by our lifestyle choices." ("AThymeToHeal.pdf," n.d., p. 149) If a diagnostic tool as sensitive as Thermography offers the ability to get to the root of the causes before the symptoms become unmanageable for the individual, then a practitioner is offered many other avenues to help in healing, while also offering an opportunity to monitor progress.

We have looked at how the body ideally utilizes carbohydrates, fats, and proteins as well as the micronutrients of vitamins and minerals and enzymes. When the balance of these elements is thrown off by disease or lifestyle choice, the body attempts to regain balance. In the process of regaining balance the body displays certain "symptoms" that allopathic medicine attempts to control and suppress. Natural Health Practitioners aim to look for the root causes of the symptoms and provide the body the necessary supports to help it heal itself. I have seen great success as a diagnostic tool for root causes using Computer Regulation Thermography and have also seen a dysfunctioning digestive tract as a major struggle for those individuals who are ailing. Therefore, the first place to support healing in an ailing individual is to heal the digestive tract. A normally functioning digestive tract enables the body to obtain the necessary nutrients.

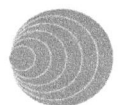

AThymeToHeal.pdf. (n.d.). Retrieved from
https://drlowdog.com/Assets/pdf_files/AThymeToHeal.pdf

Balch, P. A. (2010). *Prescription for nutritional healing* (5th ed.). New York: Avery.

Bernstein, A., & Sullivan, P. (2015, August 7). Frances Oldham Kelsey, heroine of thalidomide tragedy, dies at 101. Retrieved April 2, 2017, from https://www.washingtonpost.com/national/health-science/frances-oldham-kelsey-heroine-of-thalidomide-tragedy-dies-at-101/2015/08/07/ae57335e-c5da-11df-94e1-c5afa35a9e59_story.html

Bidlack, W. R. (1996). Interrelationships of food, nutrition, diet and health: the National Association of State Universities and Land Grant Colleges White Paper. *Journal of the American College of Nutrition, 15*(5), 422–433. https://doi.org/10.1080/07315724.1996.10718620

Biesalski, H. K., & Tinz, J. (2017). Multivitamin/mineral supplements: Rationale and safety – A systematic review. *Nutrition, 33*, 76–82. https://doi.org/10.1016/j.nut.2016.02.013

Cummings, J. H., Southgate, D. A. T., Branch, W. J., Wiggins, H. S., Houston, H., Jenkins, D. J. A., … Hill, M. J. (1979). The digestion of pectin in the human gut and its effect on calcium absorption and large bowel function. *British Journal of Nutrition, 41*(03), 477. https://doi.org/10.1079/BJN19790062

Deguchi, S., Tsujii, K., & Horikoshi, K. (2006). Cooking cellulose in hot and compressed water. *Chemical Communications*, (31), 3293. https://doi.org/10.1039/b605812d

Erasmus, U. (1993). *Fats that heal, fats that kill: the complete guide to fats, oils, cholesterol, and human health* (Rev., updated and expanded ed). Burnaby, BC, Canada: Alive Books.

Foods highest in Threonine. (n.d.). Retrieved April 2, 2017, from http://nutritiondata.self.com/foods-00008000000000000000.html

Fritchey, P. (2004). *Practical herbalism: ordinary plants with extraordinary powers*. Warsaw, IN: Whitman Publications.

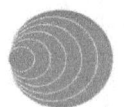

Gardiner, P., Sarma, D. N., Dog, T. L., Barrett, M. L., Chavez, M. L., Ko, R., … Giancaspro, G. I. (2008). The state of dietary supplement adverse event reporting in the United States. *Pharmacoepidemiology and Drug Safety*, *17*(10), 962–970. https://doi.org/10.1002/pds.1627

Haldiman, K., MS, & RN. (2013, June 4). The truth about stomach acid: Why low stomach acid is jeopardizing your health. Retrieved December 27, 2016, from http://thepaleonurse.com/the-truth-about-stomach-acid-why-low-stomach-acid-is-jeopardizing-your-health/

Hall, J. E., & Guyton, A. C. (2011). *Guyton and Hall textbook of medical physiology* (12th ed). Philadelphia, Pa: Saunders/Elsevier.

Hamaker, B. R., & Tuncil, Y. E. (2014). A Perspective on the Complexity of Dietary Fiber Structures and Their Potential Effect on the Gut Microbiota. *Journal of Molecular Biology*, *426*(23), 3838–3850. https://doi.org/10.1016/j.jmb.2014.07.028

Hawwa, R. H. (2015, December 25). Lysine & Threonine. Retrieved April 2, 2017, from http://www.livestrong.com/article/393914-lysine-threonine/

Hulkower, R. (2016). The history of the Hippocratic Oath: outdated, inauthentic, and yet still relevant. *Einstein Journal of Biology and Medicine*, *25*(1), 41–44.

Jaiswal, Y., Liang, Z., & Zhao, Z. (2016). Botanical drugs in Ayurveda and Traditional Chinese Medicine. *Journal of Ethnopharmacology*, *194*, 245–259. https://doi.org/10.1016/j.jep.2016.06.052

Karasov, W. H., & Douglas, A. E. (2013). Comparative Digestive Physiology. *Comprehensive Physiology*, *3*(2), 741–783. https://doi.org/10.1002/cphy.c110054

Librarian, A. a. (n.d.). Guides: Bioethics: Hippocratic Oath, Modern version. Retrieved January 3, 2017, from http://guides.library.jhu.edu/c.php?g=202502&p=1335759

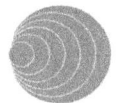
Liesha Getson. (2016). *Honoring and Empowering the Divine Feminine with Thermography*. Retrieved from https://www.youtube.com/watch?v=PJEleL8wegE

Litwack, G. (2008). *Human Biochemistry & Disease*. Burlington, MA: Elsevier, Inc.

Lutz, C. A. (2015). *Nutrition and diet therapy [electronic resource]* (Sixth edition). Philadelphia: F.A. Davis Company.

Medical-Infrared-Thermography.pdf. (n.d.). Retrieved from http://preventionandhealing.com/articles/Medical-Infrared-Thermography.pdf

Moerman, D. E. (2009). *Native American medicinal plants: an ethnobotanical dictionary*. Portland, Or: Timber Press.

Neu, J. (Ed.). (2012). *Gastroenterology and nutrition: neonatology questions and controversies* (2nd ed). Philadelphia, PA: Elsevier Saunders.

Nguyen, L. A., He, H., & Pham-Huy, C. (2006). Chiral Drugs: An Overview. *International Journal of Biomedical Science : IJBS*, *2*(2), 85–100.

Niacin Deficiency: Symptoms, Causes, and Treatment. (n.d.). Retrieved April 2, 2017, from http://www.webmd.com/diet/niacin-deficiency-symptoms-and-treatments

Pedersen, M. (1994). *Nutritional herbology: a reference guide to herbs*. Warsaw, Ind.: Wendell W. Whitman.

Petersen, C., & Round, J. L. (2014). Defining dysbiosis and its influence on host immunity and disease. *Cellular Microbiology*, *16*(7), 1024–1033. https://doi.org/10.1111/cmi.12308

Phenylalanine. (n.d.). Retrieved April 1, 2017, from http://umm.edu/health/medical/altmed/supplement/phenylalanine

Principles of Manual Medicine: Reflex Activity. (n.d.). [University]. Retrieved April 1, 2017, from http://hal.bim.msu.edu/cmeonline/autonomic/sympathetic/ReflexActivity.html

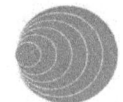

Rost, A. (1985). Diagnostik Thermoregulation. *medical focus*, *3*, 22–24.

Rost, A., & Rost, J. (1990). *Introduction to regulation thermography: practical instruction and therapeutic consequences*. Stuttgart: Hippokrates Verlag.

Rubin, T. (2015). EASY WAYS TO alkalize YOUR DIET. *Vegetarian Times*, *41*(5), 52–59.

Singh, S., Richards, S., Lykins, M., Pfister, G., & McClain, C. (2015). An Underdiagnosed Ailment: Scurvy in a Tertiary Care Academic Center - ClinicalKey. *The American Journal of the Medical Sciences*, *349*(4), 372–373.

Spinal Nerves Up Close - SpinalHub. (n.d.). Retrieved January 31, 2017, from http://www.spinalhub.com.au/what-is-a-spinal-cord-injury/what-happens-to-the-spinal-cord-after-injury/spinal-nerves-up-close

Sun, J., & Chang, E. B. (2014). Exploring gut microbes in human health and disease: Pushing the envelope. *Genes & Diseases*, *1*(2), 132–139. https://doi.org/10.1016/j.gendis.2014.08.001

Threonine Amino Acid: Structure & Function. (n.d.). Retrieved April 2, 2017, from http://study.com/academy/lesson/threonine-amino-acid-structure-function.html

Vogel, A., & Selbert, H. (1991). *The nature doctor: a manual of traditional and complementary medicine*. New Canaan, Conn.: Keats Pub.

www.ingramcontent.com/pod-product-compliance
Lightning Source LLC
Chambersburg PA
CBHW062342280526
45787CB00012B/587